DOROTHY DUSEK GIRDANO
University of Maryland

DANIEL A. GIRDANO
University of Maryland

DRUGS—A FACTUAL ACCOUNT
Second Edition

 ADDISON-WESLEY PUBLISHING COMPANY
Reading, Massachusetts · Menlo Park, California
London · Amsterdam · Don Mills, Ontario · Sydney

This book is in the
Addison-Wesley Series in Health Education

ISBN 0-201-02379-2
DEFGHIJ-AL-798

PREFACE

Drugs—A Factual Account, Second Edition differs from many of the current publications on the subject. In addition to depicting the historical, social, and legal impact of drugs on our society, it attempts to give the reader a basic understanding of the drug problem by first presenting physiological knowledge of the nervous system, and then discussing the pharmacology of particular drugs and their active ingredients, and how they relate to behavior modifications. This knowledge helps dispel the mystery about how certain behaviors such as sleepiness, alertness, anorexia, physical dependence, and tolerance occur as a result of drug consumption, and the absence of such material in many of the current books on drugs seemed to us a serious omission. It is our contention that we should attempt to understand the drug user at all levels—from microscopic nerve cells, through brain functions, to psychological and social interaction. This basic information should enable the reader to make the transition more easily from the current scene to future patterns of drug use.

To illustrate the influence of history and society's acceptance of drugs, we have included a brief historical perspective on drugs combined with some basic definitions needed for a full understanding of the drug problem. We have attempted to summarize some of the more popular reasons for drug use and abuse early in the book and to continually relate the social and cultural factors to the medical and pharmacological aspects throughout the text. Because each of the drugs of current use and interest is unique in action and effects, we have devoted a separate chapter to each drug or group of related drugs. The concluding chapters present a broad look at the use of nonprescription drugs in our society today and a summary of the ever-changing laws concerning drug use.

Because this book covers so many different topics, it is by nature general: however, the information on each of the topics is quite specific. We have selected current research which we feel best represents the knowledge amassed to date in the areas of physiological pharmacology, sociology, and psychology, and have tried to integrate the information into a meaningful discussion.

Drugs—A Factual Account, Second Edition was written to fill the needs of a wide range of individuals with different talents and interests. Fully realizing that each reader may desire further specific knowledge, we have included as many references to original scientific studies as possible. These references serve both as verification of factual information and as a guide to further research on each idea.

Additional references at the end of each chapter should also help the reader to branch out into more specific informational areas.

We hope the basic information we have supplied in this book will serve as a catalyst for continued research and greater understanding of the drug problem.

College Park, Maryland
November 1975

D. D. G.
D. A. G.

CONTENTS

1 Why Drugs? 1

Historical perspective 2
Motivations for drug use 5
Curiosity 7   Pleasure 8   Self-transcendence 9   Social alienation 10
Lack of identity 12   Apathy 12
Summary 13

2 Physiological Basis of Drug Action on the Central Nervous System . . 17

The nerve cell 18
   Transmission of the nerve impulse 18
   Drugs and nerve transmission 20
The brain and brainstem 21
   The brainstem (vital centers) 22
   The thalamus (stimulus relay) 22
   The hypothalamus (homeostasis) 23
   The reticular activating system (arousal) 24
   The cerebellum (coordination) 26
   The cerebral cortex (thought processes) 26
   The limbic system (emotional memory and behavior) 27

3 Alcohol 31

Introduction 32
Alcohol as a drug 33   Alcohol metabolism and energy production 34
Percentage and proof 41   Intoxication 43   Alcohol effects on body
temperature 45   Alcohol effects on pregnancy 45   Alcohol effects on
sexual activity 45   Cirrhosis 46
Alcoholism 48
   Treatment and rehabilitation of alcoholics 53
Alcohol terminology 60

4   Marijuana: The Great Debate 6

Introduction . . . . 6?
Cannabis . . . . 6·
Physical effects . . . . 6·
Psychosocial effects . . . . 7(
    Marijuana psychosis . . . . 7·
    The marijuana-using population . . . . 7·
Marijuana terminology . . . . 7(

5   LSD and Other Hallucinogens . . . . 7·

Introduction to LSD . . . . 8(
    Pharmacology . . . . 8(
    Physiological effects, tolerance, and dose . . . . 8·
    Neurochemical action of LSD . . . . 8·
The acid experience . . . . 8·
    LSD and spiritual search . . . . 8·
    Deceit and dangers 85
    Flashbacks . . . . 8·
    Chronic psychosis 87
    The chromosome issue 87
    LSD use in psychotherapy 89
    Creativity . . . . 9(
Other hallucinogens 90
    Mescaline (and peyote) 92
    Psilocybin . . . . 93·
    DMT . . . . 94·
    STP . . . . 94·
    PCP . . . . 95·
    Nitrous oxide . . . . 96·
Hallucinogen terminology 101

6   Amphetamines and Other Stimulants 103

General information 104
The use of amphetamines 106
    Misuse of amphetamines 107
    Weight control 107
    Physical performance 107
    Mental performance 109
The abuse of amphetamines and its dangers 109
    Paranoia and violence 111
    Psychosis 112
    Overdoses and death 112

Other stimulants 112
   Cocaine 113
Terminology of amphetamines and other stimulants 116

7   **Smoking and Health** 119

Tobacco smoke constituents 120
Motivations for smoking 122
Giving up the habit 125
The health consequences of smoking 127
   Heart disease 127
   Lung cancer 128
   Emphysema 129
   Chronic bronchitis 130
   Smoking and pregnancy 130
   Smoking and peptic ulcer 131
   Pipe and cigar smoking 131
Summary 131

8   **Barbiturates and Nonbarbiturate Sedatives** 135

General information 136
   Sedative hypnotics 136
   Tranquilizers 137
Dangers of misuse 138
   Alteration of sleep patterns 138
   Suicide and accidental death 140
Dangers of abuse 142
   Tolerance and physical dependence 142
   Treatment 145
   First-aid treatment 146
Sedative terminology 150

9   **The Opiates** 151

The opium harvest 152
The economy of heroin addiction 153
Pharmacological effects 154
Trade routes 155
History of the opiates 156
The addict 161
   Withdrawal 164
Maintenance programs 165
   Methadone maintenance 165
   Opiate antagonists 167

Synanon 168
Halfway houses and other rehabilitation centers 169
Legislative programs 170
Opiate terminology 174

10   Nonprescription Drugs 177

Sleep aids 179
Tranquilizers 181
Analgesics 182
Administration and absorption of aspirin 184
Primary pharmacological effects 184
Stimulants and antiobesity preparations 185
Other overused "medicines" 186
Regulation of nonprescription drugs 187
Nonprescription drugs as part of the drug culture 188

11   Drugs and the Law 191

Introduction 192
Philosophy of drug laws 192   Historical basis of drug laws 196
Narcotics laws 196   Marijuana laws 197   Laws relating to
hallucinogens, stimulants, and depressants 198   Possession 204
Search and seizure 205   Laws regarding drug sale to minors 205
Law-related terminology 208

12   On Being High 209

Introduction 210
The altered state 211
The drug high 212
Nondrug highs 213
Meditation 213
Biofeedback 214
Self-transcendence 216
Summary 217

Glossary 219

Index 227

WHY DRUGS?

HISTORICAL PERSPECTIVE

A *drug,* by strict technical definition, is any substance which, when taken into the body, alters the structure or function of the organism. Thus it is pharmacologically correct to call nearly any foreign substance taken into the body a drug. Because of the confusion the term *medicine* causes in discussions of drug terminology, we immediately define it here as a kind of drug—one that is taken into the body to prevent or cure a disease or a disabling condition.

Because of the development of the actual *use* of drugs (i.e., use of substance for the specific pharmacological effects they are capable of producing), we have encountered a problem of semantics in reference to drugs and drug use. This problem arises because drug use has evolved into drug *misuse* and drug *abuse*. Before attempting to follow this historical evolution, let us define *drug misuse* as the *taking of a drug for the purpose of fulfilling a need that the drug cannot pharmacologically fulfill*. Examples of misuse of drugs include taking amphetamines to improve one's athletic prowess, and taking alcohol or marijuana to improve one's social skills. There is nothing inherent in amphetamines that will make one a better athlete, nor will the two depressants cited magically change one's social skills for the better. These hoped-for reactions are beyond the chemical powers of these drugs; therefore drug misuse has occurred. Drug misuse occurs because of ignorance of a drug's effects or refusal to accept one's true motives for taking a drug.

Drug abuse can easily be defined as *repeated misuse of drugs*. This usually connotes a chronic desire for euphoria from a substance that is usually obtained illegally and carries with it a high personal and social hazard. Chronic abuse leads to socially deviant behavior and often to psychological and/or physiological dependence as well.

A second aspect of the semantic problem is related to the first, but it revolves around the *purpose* of drugs. In ancient times the general purpose of a potion was either to poison someone or to cure his ills. Our present feeling for what a medical drug (or medicine) should be has evolved from these beginnings. If an individual were sick, he took some potion to help him get well. The pattern looked simply like this:

$$\text{Sick} \longrightarrow \text{Drug} \longrightarrow \text{Well}$$

This pattern still holds for physical medicine—except, perhaps, in the case of chronic diseases such as diabetes, where once the effect of the drug (insulin) wears off, the diabetes reactions are again manifest.

This definition of a drug (what we would have to describe now as a medical drug) would still be our general definition if it were not for new psychological and social misuses of the same substances. Nonmedical use falls into this pattern:

$$\text{Sick} \longrightarrow \text{Drug} \longrightarrow \text{Relief} \longrightarrow \text{Sick}$$

In examining this pattern in relation to the first, we see that it affords no "well" end of the scale, but is instead an endless cycle. Though man has known drugs for thou-

ands of years, it has been only recently that large numbers of people have fallen
nto this kind of drug-taking cycle. An investigation of the evolution of drugs and
drug taking may shed some light on how man has arrived at this degrading cycle,
vhich threatens to continue, indeed, even prosper, in our modern society.

The change in the meaning of "drugs" and the subsequent (or consequent)
change in the reasons for taking them have been directed and redirected by the
needs, stresses, social living patterns, scientific understanding, and technological state
of all societies down through the ages. Herbs, berries, leaves, and countless other
natural plant substances were examined and used for their pharmacologic effects
from the very earliest of times. We have evidence that marijuana, a common weed,
was used medicinally as early as 3000 B.C. History tells us that as early as 1500 B.C.
the Egyptians were using opium to hush crying babies. Although some misuse and
even abuse of drugs was known at that time (marijuana was used as a cure for gout,
alcohol for pleasure), the search for drugs that would be medicinal instilled in man
the expectation of "good" from a drug because it eased physical pain. Knowledge of
drugs changed very little for thousands of years, and the concept of use was also
quite static.

The seeds of change in the concept of drugs and drug use came from such
various areas as speed of travel, speed of communication, the advent of the printing
press, scientific discovery, and the germ theory in medicine. However, all of these
stemmed from advanced technology. Technology has truly shown itself to be a two-
edged sword; as it brought comforts, so did it bring concomitant discomforts. This
may be a sign that man's ingenuity has outdistanced his wisdom—the positive feedback system of technology has created a monster that grows for its own sake rather
than for the comfort, happiness, and well-being of its creator, man.

Here are some examples of how man has allowed technology or scientific discovery to turn on him in the area of drugs. (1) The distillation process was invented
in the 800s. Before this time the only alcoholic beverages available were those having 15% alcohol or less—the products of natural fermentation. It was very difficult
to cause acute alcoholic toxicosis with a 6% ale or a 12% wine. (2) The natural
opium poppy exudate used in 1500 B.C. gave a low opiate concentration, but in
1805 science gave us a concentrated form of opiate analgesic: morphine. Along with
this milestone came the hypodermic syringe in 1834, giving us now a more concentrated opiate derivative and a method by which it could be taken directly into the
bloodstream. But technology marched on and gave us a new "hero" of analgesia,
heroin, in 1890. This new drug was of even greater concentration and carried with
it a euphoria unknown in morphine or the other opiate derivatives. (3) Man's desire
to find the "active ingredient" isolated cocaine from the coca leaf and gave us another drug that would cause a flash of euphoria. This euphoria was not possible for
the poor Peruvian Indians, who had been chewing the raw coca leaves for hundreds
of years to help cope with a rugged, sparse existence in the high Andes.

These are but a few of the drug-related scientific "advances" that have made
possible the change in attitudes toward some of the common drugs in our culture.

When we look at the patterns of technological change from ancient times till
now, we also see that the pattern of drug use has followed the overall trend of

"modernization" or technological advancement. Imperceptible advancement oc
curred before the birth of Christ through about the eighteenth century, when the firs
great eruptions of speed, knowledge, and scientific theory occurred. By the 1900
there were full-blown explosions in technology. In the late 1800s travel had bee
limited to speeds of around 100 miles an hour, but by 1940 airplanes were travelin
at four times that speed. In another 10 years their speed had again doubled. The
rocket planes in the 1960s were traveling at speeds of 4000 miles per hour—fiv
times faster than anything built a mere 10 years before. Now outer space rocket
coast along at speeds around 20,000 miles an hour. It is important to note this ex
ample of the rate of change we have experienced in our country, because the chang
in drug concepts is a close parallel.

In the late 1800s great discoveries were taking place in physical medicine. Be
fore this time van Leeuwenhoek had pioneered the use of the microscope, Fahrenhei
had developed the mercury thermometer, and the basics of chemistry and biolog
had laid a foundation for such scientists as Koch and Pasteur to postulate the gern
theory and for Jenner to discover the smallpox vaccine. Vaccines were revolutionar
in the field of medicine—at last there were drugs that could be taken to ward o
diseases that in the past had decimated entire cities. The world had waited thousand
of years for such a breakthrough, but it was then only half a century before th
sulfa drugs, penicillin, and other broad-spectrum antibiotics were developed. Thes
great events in our medical history were basic to the American feeling at the tim
that drugs were good—they cured or prevented physical debilities.

Shortly after the introduction of the antibiotics, another medical milestone wa
reached. For years we had been dealing poorly with the ever-increasing problen
of mental illness, but in the 1950s tranquilizers were first used to help the mentall
ill become a functioning part of society again. The advent of tranquilizers was im
portant for two reasons: first, the fact that we could effectively treat the mentall
ill with a drug was a breakthrough in psychiatric medicine; and second, the wor
"drug" had to take on a slightly different connotation because now medicine wa
going beyond the physical and using a drug to alter the mind.

Amphetamines and barbiturates, both mind-altering drugs, had been develope
and were being used by the time antibiotics were discovered, but at that time societ
was more concerned with physical cure than with psychological alterations. It migh
be said that these two types of drug were not being highly misused or abused a
that time because of society's definition of drugs in general.

Increased use of drugs for the euphoric effects they delivered led to new dru
terminology, for it was found that chronic users of some of these new psychoactiv
drugs did not fit the World Health Organization's description of the addict. Th
WHO described *addiction* as a condition in which the addict was committed to hi
or her drug physically and mentally, had progressed steadily along the toleranc
ladder, and was a societal problem. It was learned, however, that many of these ne
drugs did not produce physical dependence, but the mental drive to take them wa
still overpowering. Hence, the term *psychological dependence* (or psychic depen
dence) was coined. This took up where the old term "habituation" left off. It wa

xplained as a strong desire or compulsion to continue use of a psychoactive drug, a raving for repetition of the pleasurable, euphoric effects of the substance.

Once the mental form of dependence was designated, the term *physical depen-lence* also came into being. This denoted that the body developed a cellular demand or a specific drug. (The only way in which physical dependence can be made known s by taking the drug away from the user. If he develops withdrawal symptoms or he abstinence syndrome, he has become physically dependent on his drug.)

So, even though the term "addict" still conveys an adequate message, the more precise terms denoting "dependence" are preferred. Discouragement of the use of he term "addiction" may help eradicate society's stereotyped picture of the "ad-lict" as a criminal. We may then be able to treat dependence on drugs as a sickness.

We have pointed out that scientific discovery in the middle and late 1800s gave is certain elements that would later be used to the detriment of man's well-being, out before they would be so used, man had to set the stage. Unfortunately, as we broadened the capabilities of new drugs throughout the 1940–1970 "explosion" period, we were also creating a world in which our society became increasingly sus-ceptible to their effects, especially those of the psychoactive drugs.

Because of the stresses and strains of a society caught up in rapid change, the psychotropic drugs that gave us little problem in the early part of the century slowly crept into medicine cabinets all over the country to act as "sleeping aids" for an overstimulated, overanxious society and as "pep pills" for a bored, depressed so-ciety. Often both uppers and downers were found together, being used in daily cycles. And if it were not psychoactive prescription medicines that were to be found n the medicine cabinets, it was the vast array of over-the-counter nonprescription drugs that flooded the market. The use of OTC drugs probably stems from home-remedy beginnings, but the home-remedy idea has flourished into a multimillion-dollar nonprescription drug business today (see Chapter 10). Thus the drive for self-medication has led Americans from the honey-molasses-horseradish cure to the elixir to the "E-Z Sleep" to the prescription drug that in many cases can be reor-dered without a new prescription.

MOTIVATIONS FOR DRUG USE

The social and technological events of the last century have subtly determined our present-day connotation and accepted definition of drug terminology. This terminol-ogy continues to be of fluid base, dependent on our social and physical stresses and our reaction to them. To examine the motives for drug taking during the present decade is to examine the American life-style and how it is continuously changing. The 1960s saw an upsurge of drug taking in the younger segment of society and there was an immediate terminologic confrontation. The individuals taking drugs called themselves drug "users" while a large portion of the older segment of society called them drug addicts or drug "abusers." The researcher stepped in and compartmentalized drug-taking behavior: some drug takers consumed drugs every day (many of whom got high every day); another segment took drugs several times a week, but less than once a day; and this continuum finally reached those who had taken illicit drugs only once and never returned to them. From the drug surveys made by researchers, it was possible to form a composite picture of what drugs were taken, how often, by whom, and in what proportions.

In the extrapolation of data from recent surveys it appears that the majority of Americans between the ages of 16 and 25 try drugs once or twice and do not repeat the experience. (Since alcohol and tobacco cigarettes are not cited in many drug surveys, they are not included in this illustration.) Between the one-time users and those who need drugs every day lies the continuum that is described here in terms of motivation and frequency of drug use.

The triangular form in Fig. 1.1 is used to indicate the motivations that best coincide with the various frequency patterns, with the most serious (from the point of view of rehabilitation or social deviancy) at the base of the triangle and the least serious at the tip. That tip exemplifies the majority of users, since about 55% of the 16–25-year-old population report that they have used drugs once or twice and have not engaged in any further drug experimentation. The motivation for this abbreviated drug behavior is probably curiosity and requires no rehabilitative thrust. There exists in all of us an intrinsic desire to experience the unknown and this desire is especially pronounced in the ages of strong peer influence, when many of a youngster's friends are experiencing drugs. Contradictions regarding psychological effects and medical hazards that are constantly seen in news reports also enhance the desire to discover something of the unknown.

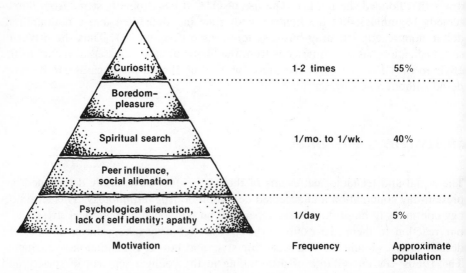

Fig. 1.1 Approximate percentage of population indulging in, frequency of, and motivation for drug consumption (alcohol and nicotine not included) in 16–25-year-old American survey respondents.

Just as curiosity is a short-term motivation in the majority of this population, it can also be an initial factor exposing vulnerable individuals to effects that will meet other motivational needs. These individuals will continue to take drugs, but with a reason more profound than that of mere curiosity.

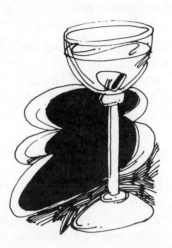

The next less serious motivation for drug taking as shown in Fig. 1.1 is that of pleasure and recreation, which can be viewed as the antithesis of boredom. The continuum between these two ends involves a variety of motives, but summarily one could say that these individuals take drugs to have fun, to escape from boredom. The frequency paralleling this motivation falls between the once-a-month to once-a-week categories.

Contemporary society has experienced an ever-increasing number of problems created by affluence, population growth, and related factors that have a bearing on drug-taking behavior. Space-age technology and rate of change have created more leisure time, which has led in turn to an apparent lack of meaningful activity and disinterest in the things about us. Instant foods, instant energy, and prepackaging have eroded the ability to endure boredom and consequently many Americans learn to expect the excitement of the "instant high."

Although our culture is expected to shoulder some of the responsibility because it creates stresses and provides forms of instant relief, each individual must learn how to deal with monotony within himself. As Bertrand Russell in his work *The Conquest of Happiness* [7] suggests, one should learn in childhood to endure a monotonous life because no great achievement is possible without persistent work. An effective antidote for monotony is meaningful activity—activity which challenges creativity.

The further we progress from the day-to-day fight for survival of our pioneer forefathers, the more time we have for less essential activity. This activity can be creative, but the problem is that far too many individuals have had increasing amounts of free time thrust upon them without proper education as to the creative use of this time. Passive forms of entertainment and excitement, devised to fill the

vast time void, give the misconception that fulfillment can be realized through activities not requiring our own energies and creativity. This then contributes to the pleasure motivation for drug taking. Like so many recent studies concerning the reasons
for drug use, an investigation by Burke [1] revealed that pleasure equals curiosity
as the reason most often cited for using drugs.

Pleasure motivation can be viewed in two ways:

1. Drugs *for* pleasure—the use of drugs at a social affair as refreshments or for the
   purpose of augmenting sociability. In this situation the social interaction is
   the main goal or pleasure being sought, i.e., the drug is a means to an end. One
   would no longer be able to enjoy the party when a disabling high developed.
2. Drugs *as* pleasure—the effect of the drug being the pleasure sought and an end
   in itself.

If either pleasure-motivation form were to become compulsive, it would depart from
the realm of recreation.

Maslow's [4] ideas on deficiency-need gratification offer insight into the pleasure motivation. If one takes a drug to overcome boredom or seek excitement and
pleasure, the drug may produce that end. However, when the high is over, the drug
taker returns to the same baseline level from which the high ascended; hence no
personal growth has occurred (Fig. 1.2).

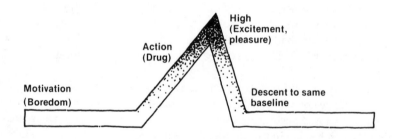

Fig. 1.2 Motivation model based on Maslow's deficiency-need gratification theory.

The antithesis of Maslow's deficiency-need gratification as a motivator is growth
motivation, which substitutes creative activity for a drug (or its parallel), and estab-
lishes a new, higher baseline, with the area between baselines called personal growth
(Fig. 1.3).

There is little question that America has and will continue to regard drugs as a
form of pleasure. Nearly 70% of our adult population drink alcohol, nearly 50%
smoke cigarettes, and 12% have "happened to have tried" marijuana (as the Gallup
people phrased their question).

Neither the mainstream culture nor the various subcultures have chosen to live
without the pleasure derived from drugs and there is little chance that such an event
will occur. Because of this fact many drug programs in the United States have been
doomed to failure, because they attempt to eradicate all drug taking rather than

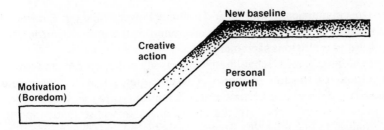

Fig. 1.3 Motivation model based on Maslow's growth-motivation theory.

concentrate on drug use patterns likely to result in drug dependence, the real drug problem [3].

True pleasure motivation is not seen here to be of serious consequence unless it is an initial step to more serious motivation in susceptible individuals (i.e., social drinking is not the cause of alcoholism).

Moving toward the base of the motivational triangle shown in Fig. 1.1, we see that the boredom–pleasure continuum gives way to an ambiguous feeling of search. The search for self-transcendence, the meaning of life, and one's reason for existence is as old as time. No one individual or group may be credited with the idea that drugs might help in this search, but mystics and certain peoples such as the Aztecs and the Indians of the Native American Church have, for years, used mind-altering

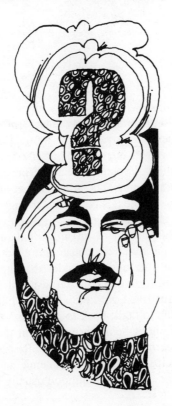

chemicals to communicate with their Ultimate Power. Chapter 5 deals with this subject in depth, providing historical background to the upsurge in the use of psychedelic drugs as a religious sacrament.

As would be expected, rehabilitative efforts are not often directed toward those who take drugs for spiritual purposes. The exception might be those zealots who lose themselves to drugs and become lost in a fantasy world that bears no relation to ongoing society. Again, these are the drug-vulnerable whose motivation has gone from spiritualism to one reflecting deeper psychological maladjustment.

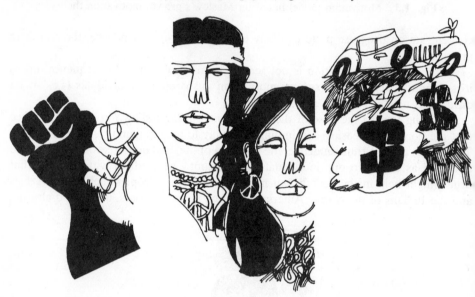

The two remaining sections of Fig. 1.1 deal with alienation and are closely related, although we will discuss them separately. The term *alienation* has been used to describe two different phenomena related to motivation for drug use. One is termed *psychological alienation,* an intense feeling of estrangement and separation not only from society's established values, but also from any subculture and often from individual goals and life meaning. The other kind of alienation is *social alienation,* which is represented in the next step in the triangle as peer influence, and further explained by theories of conformity.

Social alienation is the alienation of an individual or whole group from the dominant society. In theorizing about the cause and effect of contemporary social alienation of American youth, one might consider that many of those involved in the counterculture were reared to live out the fantasies of their parents who, while always working hard, were frustrated with the assembly line, the big organizations, and bureaucracy. Being unable to "talk back to the boss," they gave more freedom to their children to dissent without being thrown out in the cold. This is part of a system of permissive childrearing which Theodore Roszal in *The Making of a Counter Culture* [6] says equips youth with an anemic superego. The carrying of childhood fantasies and dependence into adulthood usually results in an abrupt and harsh awakening, leading to unfulfilled expectations, frustration, anger, and disappointment in the dominant social structure. In the counterculture movement of the 1960s, these thoughts and feelings served to widen the generation gap and in a roundabout way were responsible for certain patterns of drug behavior. As these young adults threw off the establishment's values, guidance, and identity, they became more dependent on the subculture, which in a cyclical pattern increased social alienation. Clothing, vocabulary, hair styles, and patterns of drug use all became part of belonging. These helped to define a group that was set apart from the established society.

Some groups are as loosely defined as the members of a student body, those who are young, or those who like a particular politician (we somehow feel that if someone believes as we do, we ought to like them). Other groups are small and sharply delineated, such as fraternity or therapy groups. Regardless of the group, to be recognized as "in," one must believe or at least appear to believe all that other members of the group do. The more attractive the group appears to the individual, the more influence the group exerts over him. Members of the group influence others and are influenced by them until attitudes and actions become more uniform.

According to theories of social conformity, peer pressure or influence is the degree to which persons or groups influence the behavior or attitudes of others. This may take the form of mere compliance, which is outward action without consideration of private conviction; or the form of private acceptance, which is change of attitude in the direction of group attitudes [2]. The formation of private acceptance resulting from group compliance is subtle and not readily discerned, nor is it readily admitted by the individual that his or her attitude toward drugs and drug-taking behavior patterns developed from the influence of peers.

The most serious consideration regarding the use of drugs which reflects peer-pressure motivation is that the weaker the ego structure of the individual, the more externally motivated he or she becomes. Here motivation may subtly shift from social alienation to one of deeper, self-identity problems; hence treatment becomes necessary for that particular individual.

In the base of the triangle shown in Fig. 1.1 appear the most serious motivations for drug taking which are also the most difficult to treat in drug rehabilitation. These are deep-seated psychological problems which may or may not have been the origi-

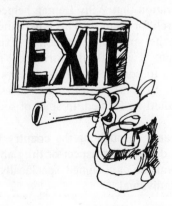

nal reason for drug experimentation, but persist as the motivation for abuse once a susceptible individual has experimented with various types of drugs. Drug takers who reach this stage have turned to the use of depressant drugs—they generally follow a pattern of alcohol and/or marijuana, then speed and/or psychedelics, and then the strong depressants such as barbiturates and nonbarbiturate sedatives, alcohol, and/or opiates. Dosages that will produce the needed high move closer and closer toward the lethal dose. The psychological motivators that are involved here are of serious consequence and deserve further exploration.

In *Love and Will,* Rollo May [5] demonstrated his insight into the prophetic nature of his neurotic patients with several examples, two of which have particular bearing on this discussion. These problems were brought to his attention in the 1940s and 1950s by his patients, people who were consciously living out what the remainder of the population was capable of controlling or keeping at a subconscious level, at least for the time being. One of these problems was that of *lack of identity,* and the other was the *inability of his patients to "feel,"* which May simply called "apathy." Both of these problems reflect what is referred to here as psychological alienation. Since the time when psychiatrists first began diagnosing these problems at an increasing rate, the endemic explosion of these symptoms has occurred just as May proposed it would, and the shrapnel still lies imbedded in American culture.

The problem of lack of identity seems to be based on changes in American society in the last several decades. Institutions such as church, school, family, marriage, and work have all undergone radical change. In May's words, "the cultural values by which people had gotten their sense of identity had been wiped away" [5, p. 26]. The role of formal religion as an authoritarian moral anchor has been altered to less authoritarian, passive preaching. The family as a centralized unit has moved toward decentralization. Sexual identity that was clearly defined in the 1950s has become much less so. Since the advent of the assembly line, fewer people than ever before see a project through from beginning to end. Impersonal mass communication and the computer have replaced much of our face-to-face contact. Thus it is not astounding that the nation has seen a rash of identity seekers, especially among the young. The institutions that had been the underpinnings of cultural values from which a sense of identity could be gained eluded not only the drug generation of the 1960s, but the parents of these young people as well. It was during the parents' generation that Willy Loman helped to trigger a realization of emptiness through his search for identity. This inheritance plus a popular laissez-faire mode of childrearing, the space-age technology explosion, and the war in Vietnam all spawned disdain, if not frank disrespect, for authority in a new generation. Heroes were hard to come by and identity was difficult to build from scratch even though Maslow, Rogers, and other humanistic psychologists insisted that a positive self-identity could be formed, in spite of social calamity, by anyone truly seeking to do so.

Drug rehabilitation research throughout the country has clearly documented the lack of self-identity as a deep-seated aspect of drug abuse, and many rehabilitation programs, such as Synanon, are aimed specifically at the formation of a positive identity within the individual.

Another psychological problem, also prophesied by May, erupted in the middle 1960s and emerged time and again in drug rehabilitation centers. This was the problem that May identified as apathy—call it alienation, estrangement, indifference, anomie, or whatever you will. This was not the social alienation of a hopeful group of "flower children," but rather the withdrawal of an individual into a lonely, hopeless inner world. To the psychologically alienated, drugs became a suicide equivalent and unless society somehow intervened, that individual would eventually subject himself to a lethal overdose.

Whether looking at these two psychological problems (apathy and lack of identity) from a prophetic or from a hindsight stance, it is clear that they dominate the drug-rehabilitation treatment efforts. They are the most difficult of drug-taking motivations to treat because therapy involves the reshaping of a personality that is as old as the individual being treated. Rehabilitation seems a misnomer in such a case, because it is hard to prove that "habilitation" preceded this state.

SUMMARY

The material presented in this chapter raises more questions than it answers. Perhaps drug abuse is symptomatic of an underlying pathology with which our society is stricken. Perhaps it is an offshoot of a new social consciousness or a backlash against bigness, depersonalization, and technology.

It is clear that society is undergoing change, and we would like to think that the current drug abuse problem is just a phase or cultural lag that we are going through until we learn to live harmoniously with chemical substances, just as we must learn to live with technology and atomic power.

If drug use is a barometer of social ills, then we must accept the challenge by analyzing the reasons for drug abuse that have been presented here and are presented throughout the remainder of this text. We must also educate young people toward the proper use of chemical substances and begin to move toward eradication of the dehumanizing patterns of our lives.

REFERENCES

1. Burke, E. L., "Drug Usage: Reported Effects in a Select Adolescent Population," *Journal of Psychedelic Drugs,* 3:55–62, 1971.

2. Kiesler, C. A., and S. B. Kiesler, *Conformity.* Reading, Mass.: Addison-Wesley, 1970.

3. Louria, D. B., "A Critique of Some Current Approaches to the Problem of Drug Abuse," *American Journal of Public Health,* 65(6):581–584, 1975.

4. Maslow, A. H., *Toward a Psychology of Being.* New York: Van Nostrand Reinhold, 1968.

5. May, R., *Love and Will.* New York: Dell, 1969.

6. Roszal, T., *The Making of a Counter Culture.* New York: Doubleday, 1969.

7. Russell, B., *The Conquest of Happiness.* New York: Bantam Books, 1958.

SUGGESTED READING

Barber, Bernard, *Drugs and Society*. Beverly Hills, Calif.: Russell Sage, 1967.

Becker, Howard S., *Outsiders: Studies in the Sociology of Deviance*. London: Free Press of Glencoe, 1963.

Blum, R. H., *et al.*, *Society and Drugs*. San Francisco: Jossey-Bass, 1969.

Blum, R. H., *et al.*, *Students and Drugs: Drugs II*. San Francisco: Jossey-Bass, 1969.

Bugenthal, J. F., *The Search for Authenticity*. New York: Holt, 1965.

Carlin, A. S., *et al.*, "Drug Use and Achievement," *International Journal of the Addictions*, 9(3):401–410, 1974.

Clark, Theodore, and D. T. Jaffe, "Studying Drug Use in the Youth Culture," *American Journal of Orthopsychiatry*, 42(2):283–284, 1972.

Cohen, Sidney, *The Drug Dilemma*. New York: McGraw-Hill, 1969.

Cowan, Ronald, and Rodney Roth, "The Turned On Generation: Where Will They Turn To?" *Journal of Drug Education*, 2(1):39–47, 1972.

DeRopp, Robert S., *The Master Game*. New York: Delta Books, 1968.

Drakeford, J. W., *Farewell to the Lonely Crowd*. Waco, Tex.: Word Books, 1968.

Ebin, D., ed., *The Drug Experience*. New York: Orion, 1961.

Eddy, John Paul, "Comment: Questionable Drug Statistics and Drug Problems," *Journal of Drug Education*, 2(1):109–110, 1972.

Glatt, M. M., *Drug Scene in Great Britain*. Baltimore: Williams and Wilkins, 1968.

Hafen, Brent Q., and Eugene P. Faux, *Self Destructive Behavior: a National Crisis*. Minneapolis: Burgess, 1972.

Herzberg, Frederick, *Work and the Nature of Man*. Cleveland: World, 1966.

Hollander, C., ed., *Background Papers on Student Drug Involvement*. Washington, D.C.: U.S. National Student Association, 1967.

Kiesler, Charles A., and Sara B. Kiesler, *Conformity*. Reading, Mass.: Addison-Wesley, 1970.

Laurie, Peter, *Drugs: Medical, Psychological and Social Facts*. Harmondsworth, Eng.: Penguin Books, 1967.

Leech, K., and Brenda Jordan, *Drugs for Young People: Their Use and Misuse*. Long Island City, N.Y.: Pergamon, 1968.

Louria, Donald, *The Drug Scene*. New York: McGraw-Hill, 1968.

Maslow, Abraham H., *Religions, Values, and Peak-Experiences*. New York: Viking Press, 1970.

McKee, M. R., "Drug Abuse Knowledge and Attitudes in Middle America," *American Journal of Public Health*, 65(6):584–591, 1975.

Mirabile, Charles S., "Psychologic Aspects of the Drug Problem," *Current Medical Dialog*, 39(3):255–257, 261–262, 1972.

Morgan, H. W., *Yesterday's Addicts: American Society and Drug Abuse 1920–1965*. Norman: University of Oklahoma Press, 1975.

Nowlis, H. H., *Drugs on the College Campus*. New York: Anchor Books, 1969.

Pope, Harrison, Jr., *Voices from the Drug Culture*. Boston: Beacon, 1971.

Post, W. H., and J. H. McGrath, "Parents and Potions—Precursors to Modern Drug Use and Abuse," *Journal of Drug Issues,* 2(1):50–56, 1972.

Rubington, E., "Drug Addiction as a Deviant Career," *International Journal of the Addictions,* 2:3–20, 1967.

Ruitenbeck, H. M., *The Individual and the Crowd: a Study of Identity in America*. New York: Mentor, 1964.

Scherer, Shawn E., *et al.,* "Need for Social Approval and Drug Use," *Journal of Consulting and Clinical Psychology,* 38(1):118–121, 1972.

Sington, D., and H. S. Klare, eds., *Psychosocial Aspects of Drug-Taking*. New York: Pergamon, 1966.

Stacey, B., *et al.,* "Drugs, Youth and Health Education," *Health Bulletin,* 32(5):216–221, 1974.

Stearn, Jess, *The Seekers*. New York: Doubleday, 1969.

Strimbu, J. L., *et al.,* "A University System Drug Profile," *International Journal of the Addictions,* 9(4):569–583, 1974.

Szasz, T. S., *Ceremonial Chemistry, The Ritual Persecution of Drugs, Addicts, and Pushers*. Garden City, N.J.: Anchor Press, 1974.

Turner, W. W., ed., *Drugs and Poisons*. Rochester, N.Y.: Aqueduct Books, 1965.

Vermes, Hal, *Helping Youth Avoid Four Great Dangers: Smoking, Drinking, VD, Narcotics Addiction*. New York: Association Press, 1965.

Way, Walter L., *The Drug Scene: Help or Hang-Up?* Englewood Cliffs, N.J.: Prentice-Hall, 1970.

Wilson, M., and S. Wilson, *Drugs in American Life*. New York: H. W. Wilson, 1975.

Wolkon, G. H., *et al.,* "The Hang Loose Ethic and Drug Use Revisited," *International Journal of the Addictions,* 9(6):909–918, 1974.

Wrenn, C. Gilbert, *Facts and Fantasies about Drugs*. Circle Pines, Minn.: American Guidance Service, 1970.

2 PHYSIOLOGICAL BASIS OF DRUG ACTION ON THE CENTRAL NERVOUS SYSTEM

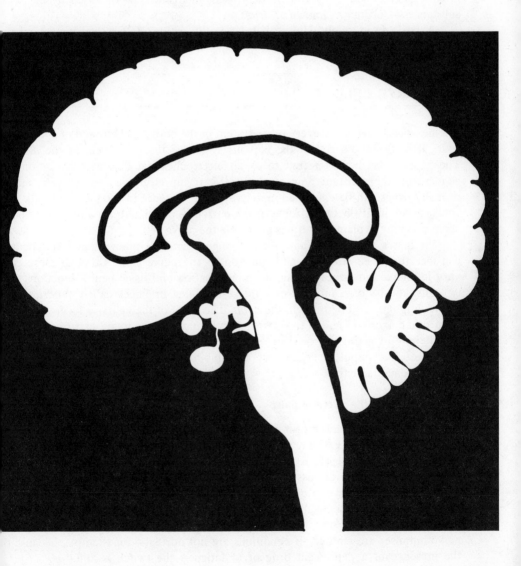

Normal function of the nervous system makes it possible for the reader to pick up this book, maneuver its pages, coordinate eyesight, be aware of the book's weight and, most important, decipher the meaning of the words, which have been arranged in statements and ideas.

Were it not for the integrative function of the brain, controlling the action of the billions of nerve cells throughout the body, neither action nor thought would be possible.

One's behavior is the result of the brain's interpretation of all incoming nerve impulses. These impulses can be depressed, intensified, or distorted by chemical substances—substances known as *drugs*.

A basic facet of the study of drugs is the action of these substances on the central nervous system.

THE NERVE CELL

The nervous system, like every other system in the body, is composed of specialized cells. The specialized cell of the nervous system is the nerve cell, or the *neuron*. The neuron has been referred to as an electrochemical unit with its action dependent on the constant flow of chemical-carrying electrical charges. The action of many drugs can be explained merely by their presence inside the nerve cell. The chemical similarity between some of the currently popular drugs and natural body chemicals may explain how drugs get inside the nerve cell.

To better understand how these foreign chemicals alter nerve cell function, consider the basic structure and function of the nerve cell. Although these cells vary in shape and size according to their location and basic neural function, they typically consist of a number of impulse-receiving branches called *dendrites* and of one impulse-sending branch, the *axon*. The body of the cell also receives stimuli from other axons (Fig. 2.1). One nerve cell may receive impulses from hundreds of different axons, some of them excitatory and some of them inhibitory. Summation of like impulses (excitatory or inhibitory) then causes the nerve cell to "fire" or remain inactive.

Transmission of the nerve impulse

A unique feature of nerve cells is that they do not come into direct physical contact with one another. They are separated by a microscopic space. This space, known as the *synapse* [5, 6], prevents continuous flow of impulses and becomes the focal point of the discussion of drug action on the nervous system (Fig. 2.2).

By analogy, the synapse serves as a switch for electric current. If conditions at the synapse are biochemically correct for the regular propagation of the nerve impulse, the switch is "on." Some drugs turn this switch on themselves and extra nerve impulses are emitted. If conditions are not normal—for example, because of the presence of a depressant drug or of fatigue—the switch is "off."

At the end of the axon (the *bouton*) there are certain chemicals located in

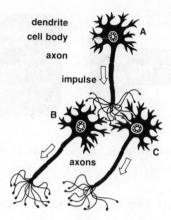

Fig. 2.1 Nerve cell A receives an impulse through its dendrites and/or cell body and sends it on through the axon. The axon of cell A sends its impulse to cell B via a dendrite and to cell C via the cell body. Cells B and C send impulses via their axons to other cells.

small pockets called *vesicles,* which appear to be all-important in transmitting the nerve impulse to the next nerve cell. These chemicals are called *neurohormonal transmitter substances.* Some of these substances that have been identified to date are (a) *acetylcholine,* (b) *norepinephrine,* (c) *serotonin,* (d) *dopamine,* and (e) *gamma amino butyric acid.* Each nerve axon contains one of these substances, produced within the axon.

The hypothesized action of this substance is as follows [4]. The incoming nerve impulse causes the vesicles of transmitter substance to join with the membrane at the end of the axon (the *pre*synaptic membrane), as shown in Fig. 2.3. Upon fusing with the presynaptic membrane, the vesicles open up and release the neurohormone into the space between the presynaptic membrane and the membrane of the next cell, the *post*synaptic membrane (Fig. 2.4).

The neurohormone has within its chemical makeup the ability to alter the postsynaptic membrane. When this alteration takes place, electrochemical reactions

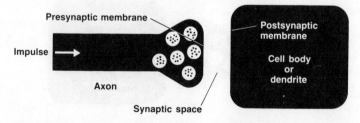

Fig. 2.2 The synapse. There is a microscopic space between the axon and the next nerve cell. The nerve impulse coming down the axon must jump the synaptic space if the impulse is to be carried on.

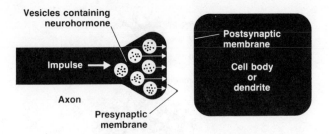

Fig. 2.3 The electrical nerve impulse causes the vesicles to move toward the presynaptic membrane.

occur which recreate a nerve impulse of the same intensity as the one that came through the preceding axon.

Nerve impulses, then, are due to *electric* current which proceeds through the cell body to the axon, where it causes *chemical* events to occur due to movement of electrically charged ions such as sodium and potassium. These chemical events at the synapse in turn recreate the electric activity necessary to carry the impulse to the next cell.

Drugs and nerve transmission

Since the synaptic events are chemical in nature, they are vulnerable to foreign chemicals, such as drugs. Looking at the synapse, consider what would happen if a drug could (a) inhibit the production of the neurohormone, (b) cause the neurohormone to be broken down more rapidly than normal, or (c) alter the postsynaptic membrane so that neurohormones would not affect it. In any of these cases, it is apparent that the nerve cell action would be depressed because there was either no neurohormone or it was not allowed to work normally [7, 9, 14]. It appears that this is the action of the depressant drugs (such as alcohol, narcotics, barbiturates) when they come in contact with nerve cells in special parts of the brain [3, 10, 21].

On the other hand, consider the drugs that cause *excess* production and release of neurohormonal transmitter substances, or have the ability to *mimic* the

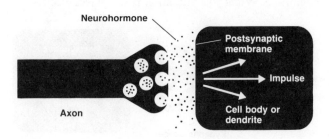

Fig. 2.4 Neurohormonal transmitter substance is released into the synaptic space and alters the postsynaptic membrane, allowing electrochemical events to occur which recreate the nerve impulse.

ction of the neurohormone or not allow its reuptake. In these cases, the neurons nvolved would be stimulated at a greater than normal rate. This is the action of he stimulatory drugs on nerve cells within the brain [14].

THE BRAIN AND BRAINSTEM

The brain controls and integrates all human movement and behavior, and nearly all drugs of abuse modify behavior by their action on the brain and brainstem. Behavior modifications caused by drugs, resulting in uncontrollable emotions, restricted information storage, limited capability for decision making, and other uncontrolled behavior, have led us to the study of how the various areas of the brain react to drugs. If one understands what events are taking place at the cellular level and at higher, more sophisticated levels, he can more easily understand why certain behavior occurs.

The brain and brainstem consist of a number of different structures concerned with the control of specific actions, thought, and emotions. Figure 2.5 depicts the brain and the brainstem down to the spinal cord. Alteration of the nerve cell transmissions within these areas affects both mental and physical behavior. Drugs are known to affect these areas, but many drugs are specific to certain structures; thus, each drug causes its own behavioral characteristics. Drug dosage is an important consideration; light doses of a drug may cause little or no behavioral change, while very large doses may cause death.

Drugs reach the central nervous system by way of the circulating blood. In general (depending on the physical properties of the drug itself), the faster it enters the bloodstream, the more rapidly its effects are felt. Drugs injected into a vein travel directly to the heart and are circulated throughout the system immediately; inhaled drugs enter the bloodstream a little less rapidly, since the chemicals involved must enter capillaries in the lungs; in general, ingested drugs take even longer, because they must first dissolve and are often mixed in with food products, thus slowing absorption into the blood supplying the digestive area.

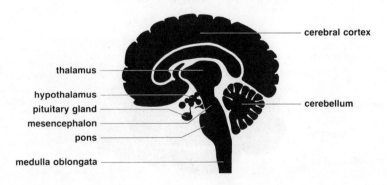

Fig. 2.5 The brain and brainstem.

Once the drug enters the nervous tissue of the brain, various effects may occur, because different drugs appear to have different target areas. Because of this specificity of drug action on the various parts of the central nervous system, the following paragraphs are designed to elaborate on the main functions of each major area of the brain and brainstem. Once this normal function is known, it becomes easier to determine logically what would happen if the action of a specific area were depressed by alcohol or a barbiturate, or if the cell action of that area were stimulated with an amphetamine or cocaine.

The brainstem (vital centers)

Medulla oblongata, Pons, and Mesencephalon. These three structures are mainly nerve fiber bundles, or tracts, that carry messages between the spinal cord and brain.

The *medulla* has special interest in that it contains the respiratory, cardiac, and vasomotor centers. When drugs completely depress this area, death occurs as a result of respiratory failure.

The thalamus (stimulus relay)

The thalamus is the "switchboard" of the brain, since all "incoming" and "outgoing" calls pass through this area.

The thalamus serves four important "switchboard" functions.

1. It serves as a transmitter of sensory impulses from other parts of the body to the sensory areas of the brain (Fig. 2.6). Specialized groups of cells do this work; these cells are analogous to switchboard operators who take incoming calls and know to what specific department (or specific sensory brain cells) to transfer the calls.

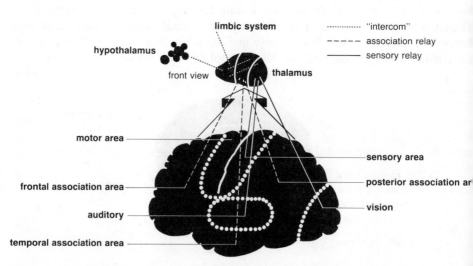

Fig. 2.6   Schematic illustration of thalamic function.

2. Another special task of the thalamus is much like the first except that the "incoming calls" are put through to the association areas of the brain. Again, specialized cell groups (called *nuclei*) send specific messages to specific brain areas (Fig. 2.6).

3. The third function is communication among subcortical areas—in our analogy this is the "intercom system." In reality, these specialized cells communicate with other thalamic areas, the hypothalamus, and the limbic system (Fig. 2.6).

4. In addition to these three functions, the thalamus serves as a relay of motor impulses back to the body.

Because of the nerve tracts, or bundles of nerve fibers, that serve as direct connections between the thalamus and the cerebral cortex, it is thought that the neocortex is the evolutionary outgrowth of the thalamus [20].

The hypothalamus (homeostasis)

This interesting structure may hold the answers to many of the mysteries concerning behavior. It is continuously maintaining body temperature, regulating the production of hormones, maintaining water balance in the body, and gauging nutritional needs, sexual needs, and countless other bodily functions.

Perhaps the two most important areas of interest concerning the hypothalamus in relation to drug abuse are those of (a) pleasure and pain, and (b) hunger and satiety.

It has been found through experimental studies that there are specific areas of the hypothalamus that elicit a quite distinctive pleasure sensation when experimentally stimulated, and there are cells that elicit pain when stimulated [8]. These pleasure and pain areas are all-important in drug use and abuse, for some drugs elicit an intense euphoria that is thought to be the result of stimulation of cells in these hypothalamic pleasure areas or depression of cells in the corresponding pain centers.

Just as there are pleasure and pain areas in the hypothalamus, it has been found that there are hunger and satiety centers also [18]. As one would expect, when hunger cells are stimulated, the body feels the desire for food. When electrodes are implanted in these areas in experimental animals, repeated electrical stimulation will cause the animal to eat itself into obesity. Conversely, if this area is destroyed, the animal will starve itself to death [17, 19]. It appears that amphetamine diet pills work on the hypothalamic satiety centers plus the pleasure areas, because they depress hunger and pep up the individual.

Integrated emotional behavior is controlled to some extent by the hypothalamus; in fact, it has been shown through animal experimentation that unless the hypothalamus is intact, fully developed rage cannot be elicited [1, 2]. Electrical stimulation of the medial portion of the hypothalamus provokes affective defense reactions, including direct attack on the object closest at hand; upon termination of the stimulation, this action ceases immediately.

In addition to controlling the emotional reaction of rage, the anterior hypothalamus appears to produce fear behavior, and stimulation of the posterior are yields alertness and curiosity [22].

Whereas stimulation of some areas of the hypothalamus has been found t bring about fear, pain, defense, and escape reactions, it is of great interest and im portance to discover that stimulation of other areas soothes an animal. Stimulatic of these areas brings about reactions akin to pleasure in experimental animal hence, these areas have been dubbed the "pleasure" or "reward" centers. Exper mentation has shown that when animals are allowed to self-stimulate this cente they often choose this self-stimulation over various delectable rewards [12]. E: perimental animals have been known to repeat self-stimulation of the pleasu center up to 4000 times an hour! However, experimental stimulation of pain cer ters can inhibit the pleasure centers; indeed, prolonged stimulation of pain cente may cause severe illness and may eventually lead to the death of the animal.

In relating the hypothalamic pleasure-pain control centers with the hypothal mic autonomic control centers (control over blood pressure, hydrochloric acid s cretion, etc.), it becomes apparent how so-called "psychosomatic" diseases migl be brought about. Chronic stimulation of pain centers of monkeys has produce ulcers in those animals.

Scientific study of drug action on the pleasure center could be very importar in studying psychological dependence on certain drugs. For example, amphetamin action on the pleasure center has been found to facilitate the self-stimulation re sponsiveness of rats [15]. Control studies showed that facilitation was due to th greater "reinforcement value" of the stimulus rather than just heightened bodil activity, which is known to occur as a result of amphetamine administration. It ha been hypothesized that the amphetamine mimicked the action of (or affected th release of) norepinephrine, the chemical transmitter substance of nerve endings i this hypothalamic area [15]. This information illustrates that amphetamines d excite the pleasure area and thus makes it easier to understand why individuals ma desire to take this type of drug repeatedly.

It is difficult to summarize the function of this underrated structure, the hypc thalamus, because it is so all-encompassing, controlling such aspects of bodily be havior as homeostasis, feeding and drinking behavior, emotional behavior, wakeful ness, sexual behavior, combinations of these, and perhaps many unknown aspect: It is beyond anyone's ability to specify detailed hypothalamic reactions to th various drugs of abuse and the human behavior resulting from these reaction: because science has not yet provided much information. However, if one applies hi knowledge of the action of depressant drugs, stimulants, or hallucinogens to th general knowledge of hypothalamic function presented here, greater insight int drug-induced behavior is possible.

The reticular activating system (arousal)

The reticular activating system (RAS) is a specialized network of cells within th brainstem (Fig. 2.7). Nearly all signals coming to the neocortex travel into th

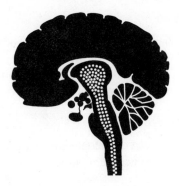

Fig. 2.7 The reticular activating system (dotted area).

RAS; that is, impulses come into the reticular formation, synapse there, and are sent on or damped out. The function of the lower two-thirds of this system is that of arousal only. Like an alarm clock, it awakens the brain (or if awake, the brain is alerted), but gives no explanation of why it has done so. Most of us have experienced awakening at night to find our covers off—sensations of chilliness synapse in the RAS and it wakes up the brain. Upon first awakening, we are not sure what is wrong. Then we assess the situation for meaning and pull the covers back on. The RAS has said "Wake up," not "Wake up, your covers are off."

In the upper third of the RAS, called the thalamic portion, the decision to send on the impulse is conditional, according to whether the message is new, different, or threatening. The ability of this portion of the RAS to damp out monotonous stimuli is extremely important to our ability to concentrate on one thing at a time. Theoretically, hyperkinetic activity denotes that the neurologic function of the hyperactive person is not up to par, i.e., unimportant signals are not damped out so that every sight, sound, smell, or other sensory input is sent on to the brain for attention. This produces an individual with a limited attention span who continually reacts to all new stimuli. It surprises many that stimulant drugs such as amphetamines or Ritalin are given to the hyperactive, but they are given in order to stimulate underactive cells of this area to produce this damping or selectivity function.

In addition to the use of amphetamines for this medical purpose, many take these drugs to keep themselves awake since the RAS is aroused by their action. The continuous activation of cells in this area by impulses from muscles, sense receptors, or stimulatory drugs will keep an individual awake and alert [3, 11]. This is the reason why muscle tension due to anxiety or fear may cause insomnia—the tension of the muscles neurologically stimulates the RAS, which in turn arouses the brain. Since the brain can arouse the RAS, worrying or thinking about what tomorrow may bring can also cause insomnia. The theories of neuromuscular relaxation are based on the importance of damping out RAS activity. Likewise, this is naturally the target of the sedative-hypnotics.

The cerebellum (coordination)

The cerebellum controls balance and coordination of body movements by integrat
ing the incoming messages from the motor area of the cortex, spinal sensory nerves
the balance system of the ear, and from the auditory and visual systems. Remova
of the cerebellum will not cause paralysis, but rather uncoordinated movement.

The cerebral cortex (thought processes)

This, the most recent evolutionary development of the vertebrate nervous system
is divided into a number of areas according to function (Fig. 2.8).

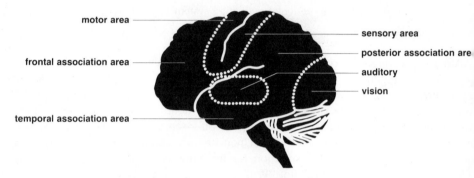

Fig. 2.8 Function of cerebral areas.

The two association areas are responsible for responding logically to time, en
vironment, and social climate. The temporal association area is involved in learn
ing processes and memory; the frontal association area is especially implicated in
drug use, since this area is the first to be depressed by alcohol and other depressan
drugs, thus removing social inhibitions [20].

The sensory area receives impulses from the body via the thalamus, and re
sponds via the motor cortex. The visual and auditory areas integrate sight and
sound into meaningful images.

Ornstein [13] has studied the role of the right cerebral hemisphere versus that
of the left side and has found that a unique control is elicited by each side. The
functions of the right and left are dichotomized into automatization and time-space
orientation, respectively. That is, the left hemisphere is highly active (and the
right hemisphere inactive) when one is writing, thinking through logic or math
problems, conducting scientific ventures, or translating and speaking a particular lan
guage. The reverse neurological situation occurs (i.e., the right hemisphere is
active and left side inactive) when one is involved in fantasy, art, dance, and music
or art appreciation. It has been suggested that drugs, meditation, and other such
highs erode the automatization through which we protect our physical and menta
being and shift us into time-space orientation. The newness of this experience and
the extension of one's ego boundaries makes right-brain dominance pleasurable
and a sought-after state.

It is obvious that drugs alter behavior, thought processes, and other reactions controlled by cortical cells. However, one general question that comes to mind is whether drugs work directly on the cortical cells, on the thalamic areas that supply information to and relay information from the cortex, or even perhaps on other brain structures that may control cerebral function, such as the hypothalamus. This must remain pure conjecture until we have sufficient scientific understanding of drug action on the brain.

The limbic system (emotional memory and behavior)

The limbic system (Fig. 2.9) is a rim of cortical tissue associated with deep rhinencephalic structures. It is phylogenetically the oldest portion of the cerebral cortex, with few direct interconnections with the neocortex, the newest portion of the brain. In drug studies the areas comprising the limbic system have often shown a high concentration of the drug and thus are thought to be effective in altering behavior. This system is in direct neural contact with the thalamus and the hypothalamus, and the latter two areas are many times included in discussions as parts of the limbic system.

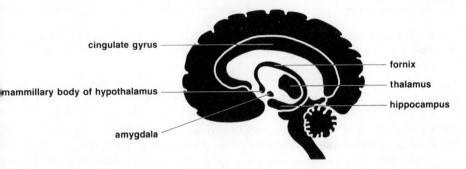

cingulate gyrus

fornix

thalamus

mammillary body of hypothalamus

hippocampus

amygdala

Fig. 2.9 The limbic system (amygdala, hippocampus, cingulate gyrus, and fornix). This system is made up of large groups of nuclei in and around the temporal areas of the cortex.

Early scientific investigation of the limbic system showed that electrode stimulation in various areas of the system would elicit changes in blood pressure, heart rate, sexual behavior, eating patterns, and many other physiological responses. This information led to a belief that the limbic system also possessed (along with the hypothalamus and other old-brain structures) specific autonomic nervous system nuclei. It is now believed that excitation of limbic areas causes efferent stimulation of lower brain centers, especially the hypothalamus, which control the various physiological responses that accompany emotion [16].

It has become apparent in only the last decade that the limbic system is the memory area of emotions. As certain situations evoke particular emotions, it is this system which provides the memory and synchronization of feelings with physiological response. If a child is afraid of the dark, this memory pattern of fear takes form

in the limbic cortex and thereafter (perhaps even into adulthood) a dark hous
or dark street, for example, may trigger this memory, complete with rapid heart
beat, increased breathing rate, and feelings of fear or anxiety. Another example i
the basis of sales techniques: good feelings derived from a successful advertise
ment may carry over into consumer behavior because a pleasant feeling is assoc
ated with the product.

As the hypothalamus is involved when one uses pleasure-producing drugs, s
too is the limbic system. If one takes a drug in a pleasurable setting or receive
pleasurable feelings from the experience, its emotional content is stored in th
limbic system and may become a stimulus to repeat the experience.

The implications of depressant, hallucinatory, or excitatory drugs in a discus
sion of the central nervous system are many and varied. There remains a wealth o
psychopharmacological information for the reader to explore; but a basic know
edge of the functions of the nerve cell and the brain should permit a greater under
standing of each drug discussed in the following chapters.

REFERENCES

1. Bard, P., "A Diencephalic Mechanism for the Expression of Rage with Special Re
   erence to the Sympathetic Nervous System," *American Journal of Physiology,* 84
   490–515, 1928.

2. Bard, P., and M. B. Macht, "The Behavior of Chronically Decerebrate Cats," i
   CIBA Foundation Symposium, Neurological Basis of Behavior, pp. 55–71. Londor
   Churchill, 1958.

3. Caldwell, J., *et al.,* "The Biochemical Pharmacology of Abused Drugs III. Cannabi
   Opiates and Synthetic Narcotics," *Clinical Pharmacology and Therapy,* 16(6):989
   1013, 1974.

4. Eccles, J. C., *The Physiology of Synapses.* New York: Academic Press, 1963.

5. Eccles, J. C., "The Synapse," *Scientific American,* 212:56–59, 1965.

6. Eccles, J. C., *et al.,* "The Mode of Operation of the Synaptic Mechanism Producir
   Presynaptic Inhibition," *Journal of Neurophysiology,* 26:523–531, 1963.

7. Grodsky, G. M., "The Chemistry and Functions of the Hormones," in H. A. Harpe
   ed., *Review of Physiological Chemistry,* pp. 426–481. Los Altos, Calif.: Lange Med
   ical Publications, 1973.

8. Guyton, A. C., *Textbook of Medical Physiology.* Philadelphia: Saunders, 1971.

9. Harper, H. A., "Protein and Amino Acid Metabolism," in *Review of Physiologic
   Chemistry,* pp. 311–360. Los Altos, Calif.: Lange Medical Publications, 1973.

10. Kopin, Irwin J., "Biogenic Amines and Drug Action," in P. Black, ed., *Drugs an
    the Brain,* pp. 3–16. Baltimore: Johns Hopkins Press, 1969.

11. Moruzzi, G., and H. W. Magoun, "Brain Stem Reticular Formation and Activatic
    of the EEG," *Electroencephalography and Clinical Neurophysiology,* 1:455–47.
    1949.

2. Olds, J., and P. Milner, "Positive Reinforcement Produced by Electrical Stimulation of the Septal Area and Other Regions of the Rat Brain," *Journal of Comparative and Physiological Psychology*, 47:419–427, 1954.

3. Ornstein, R. E., "Right and Left Thinking," *Psychology Today*, May 1973, pp. 87–92.

4. Sjoerdsma, A., *et al.*, "Metabolism of 5-HT by Monoamine Oxidase," *Proceedings of the Society for Experimental Biology and Medicine*, 89:35–38, 1955.

5. Stein, L., "Self-Stimulation of the Brain and the Central Stimulant Action of Amphetamine," *Federation Proceedings, Federation of American Societies for Experimental Biology*, 23:836–849, 1964.

6. Stroebel, C. F., "Psychophysiology Pharmacology," in N. S. Greenfield and R. A. Sternbach, eds., *Handbook of Psychophysiology*, pp. 787–838. New York: Holt, Rinehart and Winston, 1972.

7. Teitelbaum, P., "Random and Food-Directed Activity in Hyperphagic and Normal Rats," *Journal of Comparative and Physiological Psychology*, 50:486–490, 1957.

8. Teitelbaum, P., "Disturbances of Feeding and Drinking Behavior after Hypothalamic Lesions," in M. R. Jones, ed., *Nebraska Symposium on Motivation*. Lincoln: University of Nebraska Press, 1961.

9. Teitelbaum, P., and A. W. Epstein, "The Lateral Hypothalamic Syndrome," *Psychological Review*, 69:74–90, 1962.

0. Thompson, R. F., *Foundations of Physiological Psychology*. New York: Harper & Row, 1967.

1. Woolley, D. W., and E. Shaw, "Evidence for the Participation of Serotonin in Mental Processes," *Annals of the New York Academy of Sciences*, 66:649–665, 1957.

2. Yasukochi, G., "Emotional Responses Elicited by Electrical Stimulation of the Hypothalamus in Cat," *Folia psychiatrica et neurologica japonica*, 14:260–267, 1960.

SUGGESTED READING

Anthony, C. P., *Textbook of Anatomy and Physiology*. St. Louis: Mosby, 1963.

Beckman, Harry, *Pharmacology: the Nature, Action and Use of Drugs*. Philadelphia: Saunders, 1961.

Beckman, Harry, *Dilemmas in Drug Therapy*. Philadelphia: Saunders, 1967.

Biological Council Symposium, *Drugs and Sensory Functions*. Boston: Little, Brown, 1968.

Burger, Alfred E., *Drugs Affecting the Central Nervous System*. New York: Dekker, 1968.

Caldwell, A. E., *Psychopharmaca: a Bibliography of Psychopharmaca*. Washington, D.C.: U.S. Printing Office, 1958.

Chaffee, E. E., and E. M. Greisheimer, *Basic Physiology and Anatomy*. Philadelphia: Lippincott, 1964.

CIBA Foundation, *Drug Responses in Man*. Boston: Little, Brown, 1968.

Cutting, W. C., *Handbook of Pharmacology: the Action and Uses of Drugs.* New York: Appleton-Century-Crofts, 1967.

del Castillo, J., *et al.,* "Marijuana, Absinthe, and the Central Nervous System," *Nature* 253(5490):365–366, 1975.

DeRopp, R. S., *Drugs and the Mind.* New York: Grove Press, 1961.

Goodman, L. S., and A. Gilman, *The Pharmacologic Basis of Therapeutics.* New York: Macmillan, 1965.

International Pharmacological Meeting, Third, Sao Paulo, *Physiochemical Aspects of Drug Taking.* Long Island City, N.Y.: Pergamon, 1967.

Jacob, S. W., and C. A. Francone, *Structure and Function in Man.* Philadelphia: Saunders, 1965.

Leavitt, Fred, *Drugs and Behavior.* Philadelphia: Saunders, 1974.

Pines, Maya, *The Brain Changers.* New York: Harcourt, Brace, and Jovanovich, 1973.

Taylor, N. B., *Basic Physiology and Anatomy.* New York: G. P. Putnam's, 1965.

3 ALCOHOL

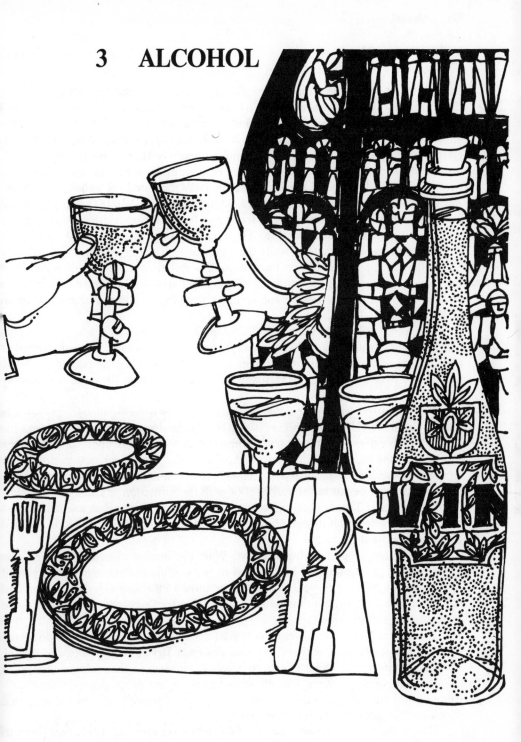

INTRODUCTION

In December 1917, the Congress of the United States passed an amendment to the Constitution which, when ratified by the necessary number of states, prohibited the manufacture, sale, and transportation of intoxicating liquors. Shortly thereafter an enforcement bill, the National Prohibition Act, or Volstead Act, was passed giving power to legal authorities to penalize severely those who produced, sold, transported, or even possessed beverages containing as much as one-half of one percent alcohol. Passage of the Jones Act in 1929 increased the penalties for making and selling liquor from $1000 and $2000 fines to a $10,000 fine plus a jail sentence. Despite these penalties, it was clear to most people from the beginning that Prohibition was unenforceable. The arrest of more than 750,000 individuals bogged down the legal system, while the worsening economic condition of the early 1930s limited the availability of the 300 million dollars needed for enforcement of the law. Since a large proportion of the population strongly opposed Prohibition and the resources necessary for enforcement were limited, Prohibition came to an end in December 1933.

Actually, Prohibition seemed to lose support from the day it was passed. This has led many historians to hypothesize that it was not really alcohol itself that Prohibitionists were against, but rather a need of one class of people to prove dominance over another. Once this was achieved, interest in the issue was quickly lost.

Drinking itself was never the central issue; it was drinking in saloons that was part of the life style of the working class. Foreign emigrants who crowded into the cities threatened the political power which at that time was concentrated in the rural communities. Prohibition was a class struggle, a political power struggle, a struggle to preserve a particular set of values, morals, and, in general, a way of life. The struggle began in the early 1800s with the formation of temperance groups in the northeast. The original appeal was religious in nature, but carried enough political power behind it to win a few local and state options; this resulted in selected Prohibition in that area.

After losing ground during the Civil War, Prohibition gained support as new organizations sprang up, and by the turn of the century the movement had spread and gained in political power. Local options turned into statewide Prohibition and officials elected on Prohibition slates finally gained enough power in Washington to amend the Constitution.

The central issue, the defense of a particular life style, was seldom discussed by eloquent spokesmen such as William Jennings Bryan, who spoke out on the harmful physical and social effects of alcohol. He argued that saloons corrupted those who frequented them, that alcohol caused neglect of family and social obligations, and that the government owed its citizens protection from dangers that they were not strong enough to resist on their own.

Unlike the Prohibitionists, the Antiprohibitionists directed themselves more to the basic issue. In England John Stuart Mill argued for personal liberty, for the right of an individual to decide for himself, for the protection of the minority viewpoint, and, at the very least, a separation of social behavior from legal sanctions. In the United States, Clarence Darrow argued that Prohibition was a diversion of attention from the real social problems not being solved by the leaders, while such labor leaders as Samuel Gompers labeled Prohibition as a means of controlling the behavior of the working class.

Whether society could not tolerate such social control or the desire to use alcohol was too great, the "wets" won out. Gradually alcohol returned to the mainstream of American life, became less of an issue, and was not considered much of a problem. More recently, however, the numerous public and private agencies established to deal with the upsurge in drug-related problems have witnessed an ever-increasing trend toward the misuse and abuse of alcohol and have sounded a new alarm. They indicate that, in reality, alcohol is the nation's number-one drug problem. Indications are that more than 10 million Americans are either alcoholics or problem drinkers whose drinking habits have adverse effects on themselves, family, employers, police, and society in general. On the average each of them affects the lives of four family members and more than 16 friends and business associates in the community. Alcohol contributes to slightly over 50% of our traffic accidents, and causes in excess of 28,000 fatalities, countless injuries, and immeasurable property damage each year. It is conservatively estimated that our national alcoholic problem costs us 25 billion dollars annually.

Although most adults and teenagers have used alcohol and are familiar with its general effects, use alone does not presuppose complete understanding of the drug. In this chapter a number of the common misconceptions and important considerations concerning the use of alcohol are itemized. The reader is asked to pause and consider each of the given statements before proceeding to the answer prepared for each item.

ITEM 1:   Alcohol is correctly classified as a drug.

Answer

Chemically, an alcohol is an alkyl group with a hydroxyl (OH) group attached. The representative of this chemical group that has produced a good deal of social and medical concern and detailed study is ethanol, or ethyl alcohol, which is contained in all commonly ingested alcoholic beverages.

Ethanol has within its structure the chemical power to depress the action of the central nervous system; thus it can definitely be classified as a mind-altering drug. With chronic use of ethanol, an individual's tolerance grows and he or she becomes physically and psychologically dependent on it.

The phenomenon of physiological tolerance to alcohol has long been recognized, though not understood. Tolerance is a condition in which it takes increasingly large amounts of alcohol to produce the same effects previously felt at lower levels of alcohol intake. Many researchers believe that alcoholic tolerance is a process of adaptive metabolism whereby the cells of the body continuously develop the capability of metabolizing increased amounts of alcohol. Other investigators suggest that it is merely a process whereby the central nervous system adapts to the alcohol that is present; that is, much of tolerance is due to the learned ability to adjust to alcohol's physical effects on speech, vision, gait, etc. Observation of day-by-day behavior of drinkers suggests that it is possible to diminish the outward signs of intoxication even though blood alcohol levels remain constant. Haymar [9] suggests that the reason for loss of tolerance in the first severe stages of alcoholism may be the permanent damage to or loss of cells that control these outward signs of tolerance.

ITEM 2:   After a cocktail a person is pepped up because alcohol in small amounts is a stimulant.

Answer

When alcohol is ingested, it is immediately absorbed into the portal venous blood and taken directly to the heart, which sends a rich supply of blood (15% of the total blood pumped per minute) to the brain. Alcohol's first effects are manifested in the cerebral area and are due to depressant action on the central nervous system.

As the tissues of the brain become exposed to the highly fat-soluble ethyl alcohol, the first cells to be depressed are those of the highest cortical areas, including the association areas of the cerebral cortex that house the centers of judgment, self-control, and other learned inhibitions. Thus, even small amounts of alcohol bring about some loss of inhibition. When learned inhibitions are removed from the government of behavior, antisocial behavior may occur because inhibitions are a result of the socialization process. As children learn to live in their society, they must learn the social inhibitions that are pressed upon them. Very early in life they learn to control their excretory processes, their tempers, and other reactions to social and physical stimuli. They learn that it is not wise to fight with older and bigger children—not acceptable, indeed, to fight at all. They are constantly being conditioned to the sexual and moral code of those around them and are expected to behave in a certain manner. As these social inhibitions are learned, they are apparently stored in the association areas of the brain as the guardians of logical, social behavior. It is obvious, then, that if these particular cells are removed, damaged, or chemically rendered inoperable by alcohol or other drugs, they will cease to guard social behavior, and the drinker will revert to more primitive behavior— the degree of reversion depending on the amount of alcohol he or she has ingested and on his or her temperament.

It is, then, this release of inhibitions that may cause the drinker to feel stimulated when, in fact, his or her brain cells have been depressed.

ITEM 3:   Alcohol causes death by overstimulating the nerve cells to exhaustion.

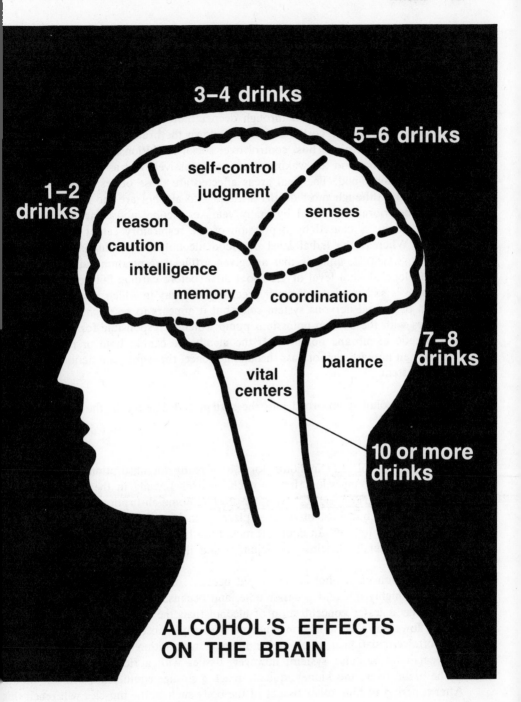

1–2 drinks
3–4 drinks
5–6 drinks
7–8 drinks
10 or more drinks

self-control
judgment
senses
reason
caution
intelligence
memory
coordination
balance
vital centers

ALCOHOL'S EFFECTS ON THE BRAIN

Answer

Even though alcohol in small amounts increases reaction time, the drug is classified as a depressant, and it is this depressant action which brings about most of the commonly observed consequences of drinking. The first noticeable effects of alcohol are due to depression of higher brain centers; as drinking continues, this depression spreads downward through deeper motor areas to the emotional centers buried beneath the cortex and further down the brainstem to the most primitive areas of the brain. Thus, control over social inhibitions, motor coordination, speech and vision, and the waking state is progressively lost as greater amounts of alcohol are consumed. The final areas affected are those of respiration and heart rate control. Although most deaths attributed to alcohol are the result of chronic physical deterioration caused by many years of alcohol abuse, acute death from alcohol toxicity is caused by depression of the respiratory center located in the medulla. Whereas the lethal level of blood alcohol in most humans is between 0.40% and 0.60%, animals that are given artificial respiration can maintain life up to a blood alcohol level of 1.20 to 1.30% before cardiac failure causes death.

There is still much to discover regarding the way in which alcohol causes depression of central nervous system cells, but it appears to researchers that alcohol interferes with the sodium-potassium pump which is responsible for setting up the postsynaptic membrane potential. If the membrane cannot hold or reestablish its integrity, an impulse cannot pass through it; hence, the depressant action on the cell and/or system.

ITEM 4: Alcohol is absorbed into the system and digested in the same way that food is.

Answer

Since alcohol is already in liquid form it is ready for absorption into the blood immediately after ingestion. It is not changed chemically in the stomach or the intestine as food is during the digestive process. Some absorption of alcohol occurs in the stomach, but most of it takes place in the first foot of the small intestine just beyond the pylorus. In contrast, most food has to pass far into the latter two-thirds of the small intestine, the jejunum and ilium, before absorption can take place.

Absorption of alcohol is very rapid because of its low molecular weight, because it is highly fat- and water-soluble, and because the bloodstream in most instances has a lesser concentration of alcohol than the stomach or intestines so it simply flows down the diffusion gradient. This rapid absorption gives the blood of the portal circulation a much higher initial concentration of alcohol than that in the remaining vascular system; however, tissues with a rich blood supply, such as the brain, liver, and kidney, quickly reach a storage equilibrium with the blood. After a period of time other tissues of the body such as the muscles will reach this equilibrium also.

ITEM 5: Alcohol has no nutritional value.

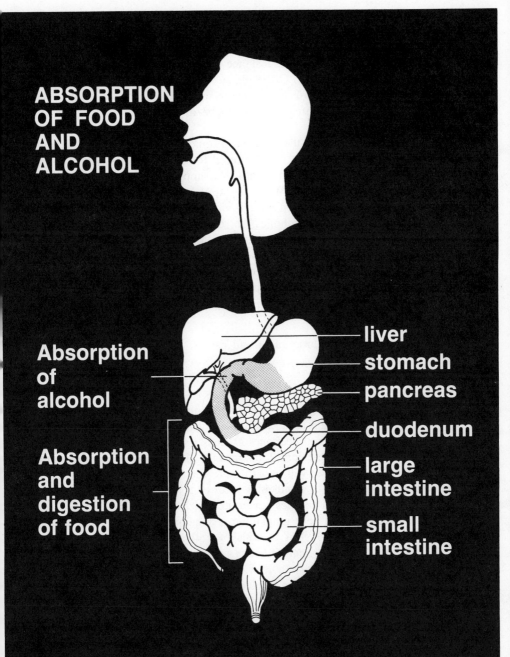

ABSORPTION
OF FOOD
AND
ALCOHOL

Absorption
of
alcohol

Absorption
and
digestion
of food

liver
stomach
pancreas

duodenum

large
intestine

small
intestine

Answer

If nutritional elements are defined as those substances necessary for the growth, repair, and proper functioning of the body and not merely energy producers, then ethyl alcohol would not be on the list of nutritive substances.

Alcohol is a highly caloric substance but contains only trace amounts of vitamins, minerals, and proteins. Often the substance that is mixed with alcohol (for example, hops and grain in beer, grapes in wine) contains some protein and vitamins, but these amounts are too small to be of appreciable value to the human organism.

The main problem in the case of chronic alcoholics is that alcohol is not merely added to the diet, but is substituted for carbohydrates, fats, and proteins. Humans usually eat in accordance with their appetites, which are normally geared in part to their caloric needs. When the appetite has been satisfied (calorically), the individual stops eating even though vitamins, minerals, and proteins may still be inadequate. In chronic alcoholics the result is often extreme vitamin deficiency that brings on polyneuritis from thiamine deficiency, fatty liver from protein deficiency, or a multitude of similar nutrition-related maladies.

In individuals who are excessive drinkers but who eat enough to meet their daily nutritional requirements, the problem is usually merely one of maintaining proper body weight because of the high caloric value of alcohol.

ITEM 6: Alcohol has caloric value and can be used like a foodstuff to produce energy in the body.

Answer

Chronic alcoholics have little difficulty maintaining energy levels even though they might consume little actual food. The calories expended for this energy come from the alcohol, which for most alcoholics exceeds a fifth of a gallon per day. Alcohol is considered to be a high-calorie food, and the alcoholic who consumes more than a fifth of whiskey per day will absorb more than 2200 calories from the alcohol alone. This may amount to as much as 75% of his normal daily intake of calories.

Alcohol yields seven calories per gram, which makes it more caloric than carbohydrates (four calories per gram) but less caloric than fats (nine calories per gram). A one-ounce shot glass of whiskey (50% alcohol) yields approximately 84 calories. A twelve-ounce can of beer (4.5%) runs a little higher at 150 calories, and a four-ounce glass of dry table wine has about 100 calories. For a more detailed listing of the caloric value of alcoholic beverages, see Table 3.1.

Like foods, alcohol must be metabolized into a chemical substance that the cells can utilize. This biochemical process begins when the enzyme alcohol dehydrogenase changes ethanol into acetaldehyde. This is the first step in alcohol metabolism and occurs mainly in the liver, although very high levels of intake stimulate at least one alternate metabolic pathway which can increase the rate of alcohol clearance. Substances that stimulate this alternate pathway can be extremely dangerous and are still to be tried in human subjects.

TABLE 3.1
Alcohol content and caloric value of various alcoholic beverages

Beverage	Alcohol content	Approximate calories
Beer (4.5%), 12-ounce can	.54 oz.	150
Highball, 1 oz. whiskey, 4 oz. ginger ale	.50 oz.	140
Manhattan, 1½ oz. whiskey, ¾ oz. sweet vermouth	.75 oz.	145
Martini, 1½ oz. gin, ½ oz. 12% vermouth	.75 oz.	150
Tom Collins, 1½ oz. gin, lemon, sugar, mix	.75 oz.	154
100 proof scotch, gin, etc., 1 oz.	.50 oz.	100
80 proof scotch, gin, etc., 1 oz.	.40 oz.	80
Dinner wine (12%), 4 oz.	.50 oz.	100
Dessert wine (22%), 4 oz.	.80 oz.	160

The first breakdown of alcohol in the liver proceeds at a rate that varies somewhat from one individual to another, but the range of variation is quite small. The average amount of ethanol that is changed into acetaldehyde is one-quarter to one-half ounce per hour. This is approximately the alcoholic content of one 12-ounce bottle of beer or one mixed drink. Within each individual this phase of alcohol metabolism is quite uniform and little can be done to speed up the process. There are some individual differences in the amount of alcohol that can be stored in the body (see Item 12), but sooner or later this stored alcohol must be metabolized. Until that time, alcohol will continue to affect the central nervous system. Since the first phase occurs in the liver at a constant rate, the process of "sobering up" is dependent on the liver. This concept is extremely important for individuals who must drive or perform other activities after drinking.

The second phase of alcohol metabolism, that of oxidation of acetaldehyde into acetic acid, takes place not only in the liver, but also in many cells of the body, including the cells of the brain and nervous system. The rate of this oxidation is very important because the accumulation of large amounts of acetaldehyde in the cell can have adverse effects on normal cell function.

Acetaldehyde serves as a substrate for several enzymes. Under normal circumstances, it is metabolized rapidly and does not interfere with cell function. However, the large amounts of acetaldehyde that accumulate after ingestion of large quantities of ethanol are significant in the development of headaches, gastritis, nausea, dizziness, and other symptoms, which, when they occur together, are commonly known as a "hangover" [10].

The problem of the accumulation of acetaldehyde is compounded by the effects of alcohol on cellular metabolism. Ethanol is a general depressant of several endocrinological processes and associated metabolic events. This decrease in general metabolism also slows down the rate at which acetaldehyde is utilized [6].

The third phase of alcohol metabolism is the energy phase, where the metabolite acetic acid enters into the normal chemistry of energy production. It is chemically changed into acetyl coenzyme-A and is used in the Krebs cycle to produce energy, just as other foodstuffs are (Fig. 3.1). When alcohol is in the system it is used preferentially for fuel, leaving the foodstuffs to be stored as fat. With this a two-fold problem occurs, one of gained weight and the other of an accumulation of fats that are not removed from the liver. The latter is instrumental in the liver disease that is seen in chronic drinkers.

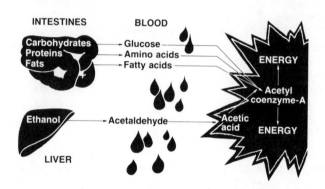

Fig. 3.1   Energy production from food and alcohol.

ITEM 7:   The "morning-after" headache from alcohol can be avoided by eating high levels of carbohydrates the night before.

Answer

The nausea, headache, gastritis, dizziness, and vomiting that often accompany excessive consumption of alcohol appear to be caused not only by high alcohol concentration in the blood, but also by the increased amounts of acetaldehyde in the tissues. Accumulation of excess amounts of alcohol and acetaldehyde further depresses metabolic activity, thus increasing the amount of lactic acid and acetic acid in the body. Large amounts of lactic acid diminish alkali reserves and the alkali-binding power of the blood. Thus, impaired respiratory exchange, which decreases normal elimination of lactic acid and carbon dioxide, combines with increased acid accumulation due to decreased alkali-binding power to accentuate the symptoms of the hangover [10].

There remains some controversy as to the value of food substances in speeding up the oxidation of alcohol and the elimination of acetaldehyde and lactic acid buildup. Proteins have been shown to speed up metabolism of alcohol in individuals whose metabolism is not at a maximum. A diet low in protein will tend to diminish the metabolic rate through depletion of the enzymes necessary for alcohol metabolism. Diets high in either fat or carbohydrates have not been shown to have any significant effect on the rate of metabolism of alcohol. Investigators have found some increases when glucose or insulin was given, but these increases occurred only in individuals who exhibited a lower-than-maximum alcohol metabolism [23]. It can be generally concluded that individuals with normal alcohol metabolism cannot increase this metabolism by prior consumption of any dietary substance.

ITEM 8:   Drinking black coffee speeds the sobering-up process.

Answer

The practice of drinking black coffee to aid in the sobering-up process has been followed for many years. However, as was shown in Item 6, sobering up or regaining control of the cells depressed by alcohol is entirely dependent on the breakdown of alcohol by the liver.

The caffeine contained in coffee is a stimulant and slightly increases the activity of cells in the central nervous system. While caffeine may or may not alleviate the intoxication symptoms, it does not speed up metabolism of alcohol. It is generally assumed that alcohol metabolism is independent of overall metabolism and is not sensitive to the overall metabolic demands of the body. Conditions such as hyperthyroidism, physical activity, or exposure to low temperatures (all of which are capable of doubling overall metabolism) have little, if any, effect on the metabolism of alcohol and on the sobering-up process [15].

Even though drinking coffee does not actually speed the sobering-up process, it still remains a sound practice so long as its effects are not overrated. The caffeine in the coffee is a central nervous system stimulant and may temporarily act as a partial stimulant to some cells depressed by alcohol. This may give the depressed person somewhat of a lift. And since sobering up is a function of time, the time spent in drinking the coffee may be of even more value!

ITEM 9:   One becomes intoxicated faster on rum or gin than on bourbon.

Answer

If the same amount of equal-proof liquors is drunk in the same manner, one liquor is no less intoxicating than the other. As was noted previously, we are speaking of one basic substance, ethanol. Whether it is distilled from fermented molasses, as rum is, or from fermented grains, as bourbon is, makes little difference. However, if the proof of one beverage is higher than another, the beverage with the higher proof will be more highly intoxicating if both are drunk in equal quantities: two ounces of whiskey is more intoxicating than two ounces of beer.

In the same vein, there is a common belief that mixing certain alcoholic beverages in certain ways will make one ill—"beer on whiskey, mighty risky"—whereas a different drinking pattern of the same drinks will not cause illness—"whiskey on beer, nothing to fear." Switching drinks throughout an evening may cause nausea, but probably more because of the amount drunk than because of the kinds consumed or the order of consumption.

The proof of a distilled beverage is its alcohol content and is roughly twice the given alcohol percentage (100 proof equals about 50% alcohol). A 100-proof spirit is an alcoholic beverage in which the alcohol has a specific gravity of 0.93426 at 60°F. This is the weight of the substance per volume compared to the weight of the same volume of water. It is said that in the early testing of alcoholic beverages the distiller mixed his whiskey with gunpowder, and if the alcohol content was too low the mixture would not light. If the whiskey was too strong, the gunpowder

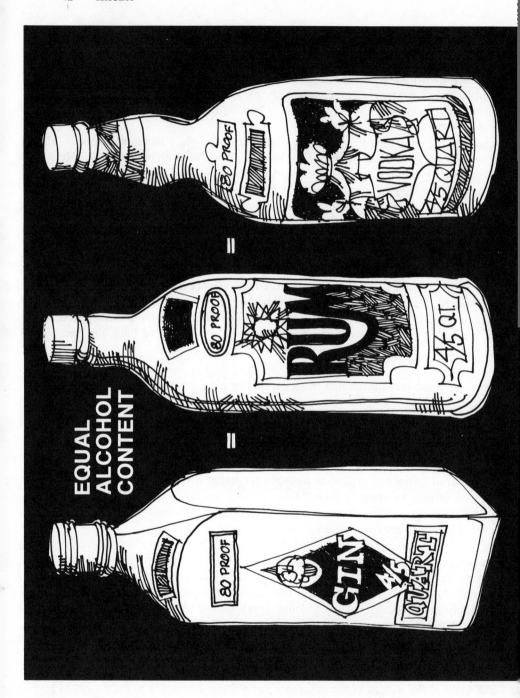

amed up wildly. But if the alcohol content was near that desired, it would burn with an even, bright blue flame. This kind of flame was "proof" of good whiskey [1].

The proof, or percent alcohol, of a drink should be of concern to everyone who drinks or serves alcoholic beverages, so that he can intelligently judge the pacing of his drinks and the proper waiting period before he drives or takes on some other responsibility. As was pointed out earlier, the alcohol contained in one cocktail or a 12-ounce bottle of beer is oxidized in approximately one hour. For a listing of the alcohol content in various alcoholic drinks, see Table 3.1.

ITEM 10: One cocktail is not likely to greatly impair driving ability.

Answer

Although individuals differ in their reactions to ingested alcohol, one cocktail is usually not likely to interfere with one's driving skill. For instance, a small person drinking a cocktail on an empty stomach may be adversely affected by that drink, but for most people the approximate blood alcohol content (0.02% to 0.03%) resulting from one cocktail is not high enough to make a difference in driving ability.

Blood alcohol levels are given in milligrams of alcohol per 100 milliliters of blood: If a person had 50 mg of alcohol per 100 ml of blood, he would have a blood alcohol content of 0.05%. Roughly speaking, four to five ounces of whiskey in the average individual (154 pounds) ingested over a period of one hour would give a blood concentration of about 0.10% in two hours.

It is generally found that at a blood alcohol level of 0.02% there is no discernible intoxication. Between the levels of 0.05% and 0.09% there are various signs of intoxication, but these levels would not be legal proof of drunken driving in most states. Most individuals are, however, unmistakably drunk at a level of 0.15%, and at a level of 0.3% *any* drinker would be intoxicated. At 0.45% intoxication is severe and further ingestion of alcohol could well result in death; indeed, levels as low as 0.35% to 0.45% have been known to cause death. Levels above 0.55% are usually fatal in untreated patients. For a thorough summary of the effect of various levels of blood alcohol concentration, see Table 3.2.

ITEM 11: If an individual has a blood alcohol level of 0.15%, he or she could be arrested for driving while intoxicated in any state in the United States.

Answer

At 0.15% a driver would be considered legally intoxicated in all states of the United States in accordance with the original criterion set up by the National Safety Council. However, this agency more recently advocated a legal intoxication level of 0.10% and virtually all states have complied. Utah has the lowest minimum, 0.08%.

ITEM 12: An obese 250-pound individual should be able to "hold his liquor" better than a muscular individual of the same weight.

TABLE 3.2
Psychological and physical effects of various blood alcohol concentration levels

Number of drinks†	Blood alcohol concentration	Psychological and physical effects
1	.02–.03%	No overt effects, slight feeling of muscle relaxation slight mood elevation.
2	.05–.06%	No intoxication, but feeling of relaxation, warmth Slight increase in reaction time, slight decrease in fine muscle coordination.
3	.08–.09%	Balance, speech, vision, and hearing slightly impaired. Feelings of euphoria. Increased loss of motor coordination.
4	.11–.12%	Coordination and balance becoming difficult. Distinct impairment of mental faculties, judgment, etc.
5	.14–.15%	Major impairment of mental and physical control Slurred speech, blurred vision, lack of motor skill Legal intoxication in all states (.15%).
7	.20%	Loss of motor control—must have assistance in moving about. Mental confusion.
10	.30%	Severe intoxication. Minimum conscious control of mind and body.
14	.40%	Unconsciousness, threshold of coma.
17	.50%	Deep coma.
20	.60%	Death from respiratory failure.

* For each one-hour time lapse, subtract .015% blood alcohol concentration, or approximately one drink.
† One drink = one beer (4.0% alcohol, 12 oz.) or one highball (1 oz. whiskey, 4 oz. ginger ale).

Answer

Being able to "hold one's liquor" depends on a variety of circumstances: (a) the presence of food in the stomach, (b) the rate of consumption of alcohol, and (c) the concentration of the alcohol. Food, especially milk, fats, and meat, slows the absorption of alcohol. This allows more time for alcohol metabolism to proceed Obviously, the rate of alcohol consumption is important, for if large amounts are consumed in a very short time, the concentration of alcohol in the stomach and intestine would cause rapid absorption. However, concentrations of alcohol above 50% (that is, beverages that are more than 100 proof—unusually strong) often exert a depressant effect on absorption. This may be due to a depression of stomach movement which delays emptying of stomach contents into the intestine; or it may be that the high concentration of alcohol irritates the mucosal lining of the stomach and intestine, causing an increase in the secretion of mucus, and thus delaying absorption.

On the other hand, alcohol diluted to 10% or less, as in highballs, is absorbed slowly. The most rapid absorption usually occurs with wines and stronger mixed drinks such as martinis and manhattans, in which the percentage of alcohol is somewhere between 10% and 40%. Under most conditions the drink with 40% alcohol would be absorbed more rapidly than the one with 10% because of the normal concentration gradient [10].

After alcohol is absorbed from the stomach or intestine, it passes into the portal system and is distributed throughout the body. When the blood alcohol level exceeds that of the tissues, alcohol is absorbed into the tissues and exerts its depressant effect there. Even though muscle tissue absorbs alcohol, the resulting depression of muscular activity is minor; the muscle tissue, in effect, stores the alcohol. Alcohol is not absorbed in fat tissue to the same degree as in muscles, probably because of the low water and protein content of fat. The 250-pound individual with a high fat content lacks the storage advantage of muscle tissue; consequently, more alcohol is left to affect the nervous system than is the case with a muscular individual.

ITEM 13: At a cold football game it makes sense to drink alcohol because alcohol increases body temperature.

Answer

The effect of alcohol on the vascular system is one of mild dilation of the peripheral blood vessels (those nearest the skin), with an accompanying slight drop in blood pressure. This vasodilation occurs as a result of depressive action on the vasoconstrictor centers in the medulla (this action may be mediated by a higher brain center such as the hypothalamus). The normal state of these vessels is a constant vasoconstriction; thus, when alcohol dulls the cells which emit constrictive impulses, the vessels relax and become dilated. When the peripheral vessels are enlarged, more blood is allowed to flow to the peripheral areas of the body, where it comes in close contact with the external environment. If the external environment is cooler than body temperature, heat will be lost from the body. With a greater amount of blood flowing to the peripheral areas of the body, body heat loss occurs more rapidly. Therefore, even though a football game spectator may feel a warm flush after drinking an alcoholic beverage, he or she is actually causing a decrease in body temperature.

ITEM 14: An unborn child is not affected by its mother's consumption of alcohol.

Answer

Any drug that enters the bloodstream of a pregnant woman soon reaches the placenta, often in highly undiluted form. Many soluble materials are capable of crossing the placenta, entering the fetal bloodstream, and chemically acting on fetal structures. Alcohol is one of these substances.

The pregnant mother, by virtue of her adult status, has the ability to detoxify her body by breaking down foreign substances, but the unborn fetus has a number of handicaps that leave it much more vulnerable to a toxic drug. These handicaps are as follows:

1. The fetus has the anatomical disadvantage of an enormous surface area of placenta villi, which permits easy transfer of such a substance as alcohol from the mother's blood to the blood of the fetus.
2. Its gastrointestinal mucous membrane has a high degree of permeability.
3. The fetus is deficient in functional kidney structures (glomeruli), which help excrete unwanted substances from the body.
4. Fetus enzyme systems are insufficiently developed to effectively break down or metabolize foreign substances.

Thus, until the fetus leaves its uterine environment, its ability to metabolize or detoxify toxic substances is hampered.

Because it is unfeasible to do experimental work on human fetal reactions to alcohol, it is quite impossible to state exactly what the reactions are, but an understanding of alcohol's effects on the adult enables one to theorize on fetal effects. When alcohol reaches the cells of the fetus, it must surely depress cellular action and interfere with normal processes there, just as in the adult.

A mother who is intoxicated during delivery will give birth to a child who is, to a degree, also intoxicated (depending on the amount of alcohol the mother has consumed). Indeed, a child born to an alcoholic mother may have to be gradually withdrawn from alcohol just as a child born to an opiate addict must be withdrawn from that drug.

ITEM 15:   Alcohol is an aphrodisiac.

Answer

Though cordials and liqueurs are no longer thought of as love potions, it is interesting that nearly all the basic ingredients of the common liqueurs can be found listed in Arab, Chinese, and Hindu "recipes" for aphrodisiacs, those supposedly magic, mystical stimulants of the libido.

Through the years, alcohol has been called the "handmaiden of Cupid" not because of its stimulant effect on sexual desires, but because its suppression of inhibitions causes some reluctant females to become more agreeable in romantic matters. Adams [1] would aptly quote here the old saying, "Some girls are cold sober, others are always cold."

Sexual functions are basic to life and thus, like breathing, eating, and drinking, have their origin in what is commonly called the "old brain," or the midbrain. As the civilized world developed the "new brain," or cerebral cortex, it took over the control of sexual functions, elimination processes, etc., so that no longer did humans react immediately to basic desires, but learned to put these desires into a logical, thought-inspired perspective that generally satisfied the society in which they lived.

After ingestion of alcohol, a drinker may react to basic sexual stimuli in a way ı which he or she would not normally react, because alcohol has diminished erebral inhibitions.

However, as a person continues to drink, his or her actual sexual prowess or ability to perform" diminishes because of loss of neural control and coordination.

ГЕМ 16: Alcohol's direct effect on the liver is the main cause of the high incidence f cirrhosis among alcoholics.

ınswer

ـaennic's cirrhosis is a chronic disease in which there is a progressive spread of onnective tissue between portal spaces where there was once functional tissue. It ; believed to develop by a process of fat accumulation followed by dysfunction and ınally by fibrosis of the liver. It is also theorized that hepatitis may be a step in his disease process.

About 75% of all alcoholics show impaired liver function and approximately ;% of all alcoholics eventually develop cirrhosis, a rate of incidence that is about ix times that of the nonalcoholic population. Cirrhosis has become the fourth lead-ng cause of death between the ages of 25 to 45 in large urban areas.

The cause of cirrhosis has not been specifically pinpointed and a strong con-roversy among medical researchers has developed concerning this topic. Two nain theories are proposed:

1. That alcoholics tend toward malnutrition and this lack of nutritive elements allows the cirrhotic process to occur, and

2. That alcohol itself (in the presence of adequate nutrition) causes cirrhosis.

3oth theories are reasonable and merge on one major point—that fatty liver de-velops as a first step in cirrhosis.

Many attempts have been made to produce cirrhosis in experimental animals ›y feeding them alcohol, but these experiments have been highly unsuccessful. It ıppears that although the addition of alcohol to the diets of animals does not lead o cirrhosis, it does aid the hepatotoxic effects of other substances such as chloro-orm or carbon tetrachloride, and will exacerbate a cirrhotic condition that is al-eady present in an animal [10]. These studies have been criticized for not ap->roaching the alcohol concentration that alcoholics attain daily.

The basis of the malnutrition theory of cirrhosis causation is that dietary leficiencies, especially a deficiency of proteins, result in a low level of lipotropic ıubstances (such as choline, folic acid, and cynanocobalamin or vitamin B_{12}), vhich are necessary for normal removal of fat from the liver. When these lipotropic ıubstances are withheld from the diet of experimental animals, fatty liver results, ınd in most species cirrhosis follows. High-protein diets, especially those that in-:lude choline, will aid in the arrest of the cirrhotic process [17].

Fatty liver is a logical forerunner of a fibrotic condition because

a) excess fat interferes with normal metabolism in hepatic cells, thus causin death of the cells;

b) fat-filled cells next to each other tend to merge, thus creating a larger, non working complex that ruptures;

c) excess fat causes a diminution of reproductive activity in hepatic cells, an as a result, worn-out cells are not replaced as quickly as they would b normally; and

d) fat obstructs normal blood flow in the liver cells, resulting in anoxia (oxyge deficiency) and death of the cells. Once liver cells die, the fibrotic proces begins and will continue as more cells die. This is not a reversible process.

It has been shown that very high alcohol consumption also has a direct dele terious effect on the liver and cannot be dismissed as a causative agent in cirrhosis When the liver is forced to metabolize very large amounts of alcohol, there is a excess buildup of metabolites there that inhibits the production of energy from dietary fats. That is, the liver preferentially produces energy from alcohol rathe than from other foods [16]. This leads to deposition of fat in hepatic cells an holds much the same potential for liver damage as does fat deposition caused b dietary deficiency. Lieber and DeCarli [18] have recently produced cirrhosis i baboons even when there was no dietary deficiency. However, until this controvers is settled, both theories must be entertained.

ALCOHOLISM

Alcoholism is a general term describing a whole set of physical, psychological and sociological conditions, yet is specific enough to be used as a name for "drinking disease." Alcoholism in the following discussion will be viewed mainl as a medical and psychological problem, in other words, drinking that has becom pathological, chronic, and progressive, with true addictive aspects. It is well know that alcoholism does not start on one specific day in a long number of drinkin days, but rather at some point when the chronic drinker can no longer control hi or her appetite for, or use of, alcohol.

Approximately 75% of American adults of drinking age and approximately 80% of high school students have consumed alcohol. Surveys indicate that one half of the teenagers who drink do so at least once a month, but no accurate breakdown into specific frequency categories has been made for this age group In the adult drinking groups approximately 9% are classified as heavy drinkers 18% as moderate, 31% as light, and 42% as abstainers and infrequent drinkers As has been discovered about other drugs, consumption of alcohol is slightl higher on the east and west coasts and lowest in the southern states.

Characterizing alcoholics and problem drinkers or those most likely to be come so in terms of age, sex, ethnic background, religious affiliation, education geographic location, etc., is difficult and fraught with exceptions, but a compilation

f surveys by the Alcohol, Drug Abuse and Mental Health Administration [22]
eports the following profiles:

Profile of persons with high problem rates

Male, of lower socioeconomic levels
separated, single, and divorced persons
Persons with no religious affiliation, followed by Catholics and liberal Protestants
Those with childhood disjunctions
Beer drinkers, as opposed to hard liquor drinkers
Persons who believe that drunkenness is not a sign of irresponsibility
Residents of large cities

Profile of those most likely not to have alcohol-related problems

Women   Residents of southern states
Persons over 50   Wine drinkers
Widowed or married   Persons with postgraduate education
Jewish religious affiliation
Rural residents

ITEM 17:   Social drinking is the first step toward alcoholism.

Answer

This question must be considered true (but facetiously so) because, as will be
pointed out in the answer to Item 18, alcoholics generally begin their drinking as
social drinkers; however, it is most important to point out that social drinking in
itself is not the *causative* factor in alcoholism, just as matches are not the cause
of forest fires.

Social drinking does provide a "legitimized" stage for learning and fostering
drinking behavior. Approximately 75% of the drinking-age population use alcoholic beverages to some extent, and most of this drinking is done socially. With the
necessary deference given to "pot parties," the drinking party is still the most
popular drug get-together with youthful drug users. Some surveys indicate that as
many as 50% of high school students attend drinking parties at least once a month
and that half of that percentage get "bombed" once each month. At this age, peer
pressure is an important motivator, and the amount and type of beverage consumed is influenced most by one's drinking companions. For example, distilled
beverages are consumed more with friends at parties than with one's family, and
more is consumed in the presence of close friends and work companions than at
social meetings with, say, people from the church.

Socal drinking is an important phenomenon because the drinker generally
takes his or her first drink for purely social reasons. Many, however, find that the
drug meets a need and continue to take that drug for the subsequent meeting of
psychological needs. In this way, social drinking is implicated in problem drinking
and alcoholism.

ITEM 18:   Alcoholics tend to follow a general pattern of behavior on their way t alcoholism.

Answer

Apparently, the most difficult part of recovery for an alcoholic is to identify th problem in his or her mind. It has been said that the alcoholic is always the las to know that he or she is a true alcoholic. Others usually see the problem develop ing by observing the following symptoms in the drinker: being intoxicated at work having been "bombed" at least four times during the past year, driving while in toxicated, having a serious accident because of intoxication, being arrested be cause of an alcohol-related problem, or performing acts while intoxicated that th individual would not perform while sober. With this in mind, a thorough study c alcoholics was undertaken by Dr. E. M. Jellinek [14]. He interviewed over 200 alcoholics and found a characteristic pattern that constituted the "road to alco holism." With a knowledge of this characteristic pattern, problem drinkers ma recognize their problem earlier and control their drinking habits before the hab controls their lives.

The phases that most alcoholics follow appear to go from controlled socia drinking to complete alcohol addiction. These phases can be summed up as fol lows.

PRE-ALCOHOLIC PHASES

1. Controlled social, cultural drinking. The first phase is that of controlled socia or cultural drinking. It is said that some drinkers become alcoholics with thei first drink, but complete loss of control to alcohol usually progresses over a perioc of 10 to 20 years or longer.

2. Occasional escape from tensions. Just as social drinkers do not become alco holics overnight, they also have no warning that their drinking has gone beyonc that of social or cultural drinking and has progressed to a purposeful drinking—tc escape from tensions. About 20% of the nation's drinkers fall into this category

3. Frequent escape drinking. The third phase is entered as innocuously as wa the second. As drinkers find that they can temporarily escape the tensions anc frustrations of their everyday lives through the use of alcohol, they begin to turn to this escape from real life more often.

During these first three stages, the drinker's tolerance to alcohol steadily in creases, but in phase 3 alcohol tolerance takes a sharp upswing and he or she mus drink more and more liquor to achieve the same nirvana that was previously ex perienced (see Fig. 3.2).

EARLY ALCOHOLIC PHASE

4. A progression of drinking takes the escape drinker into the fourth phase, which appears to begin with the occurrence of the first blackout. The blackout is not merely passing out from drinking too much, but is more like temporary am-

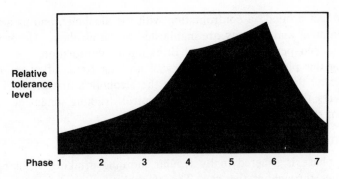

Fig. 3.2 Tolerance to alcohol during characteristic phases of alcoholism. (Modified from Jellinek, 1952, p. 67.)

nesia. One may carry on a conversation, move about, even drive his or her car—but will remember none of these actions later. It has been hypothesized that this phenomenon is due to the drinker's willpower—he or she wishes to remain in control of his or her body to prove that he or she can handle the liquor, but the drug effect still overtakes part of the brain so that memory patterns are not established.

Tolerance continues to develop slowly during this phase and will continue through phase 5, where it reaches its peak.

The actions of problem drinkers during this phase may be characterized as a progressive preoccupation with alcohol. When social functions are announced, they are more interested in whether drinks are to be served than in who will be attending the function. Before attending social functions, they fortify themselves with alcohol, and at parties they are in continual pursuit of an alcohol supply. This drinker is far past the social drinking stage. He or she may begin to drink alone, gulping down the first few drinks to obtain an immediate effect, and his or her behavior may begin to be embarrassing to others, especially the husband or wife of the drinker. Also, during this phase, problem drinkers may develop conscious or unconscious guilt feelings about their drinking and offer "good excuses" for taking a drink. No longer do they brag about their alcohol consumption, but rather tend to underestimate the number of drinks they have consumed. They begin to avoid conversation concerning alcohol altogether.

At this time changed drinking patterns (drinking at a different time of day, switching to a new alcoholic beverage, using a different mix, etc.) may be used as a means of controlling one's drinking habits, and there may even be periods of total abstinence to prove that alcohol is still on a "take-it-or-leave-it" basis.

TRUE ALCOHOLIC PHASE

5. Again, let it be emphasized that these phases are not definite periods of time made obvious by calender dates or road signs. Over a period of time chronic drinkers move from the early alcoholic stage to the true alcoholic phase, in which everything in their being revolves around alcohol. Appearance, home relations, job, and possessions are neglected and begin to deteriorate. Family members change their habits to "get around" a confrontation with the alcoholic, and as a result of this, deep resentment and self-pity are manifested in the alcoholic. He or she may go through extended periods of constant drinking for consolation.

It is during this phase that the drinker can no longer stop after one drink. It has been suggested that perhaps by this time the alcoholic's first drink of the day or evening affects those cortical cells which control drinking judgment, and thus he or she cannot stop after one drink.

COMPLETE ALCOHOLIC DEPENDENCE

6. The sixth phase is ushered in by regular morning drinking, drinking which usually continues throughout the day. The alcoholic is now in danger of withdrawal symptoms if alcohol is not kept in his or her system at all times.

This phase is often represented by the comic figure who hides bottles all over the house and office. But at this point the alcoholic is really a tragic figure, who neglects proper nutrition and whose family life deteriorates to the point of complete disruption. Alcohol is the alcoholic's purpose for living; he or she has become totally addicted to this drug.

7. The last phase of alcoholism is one in which social, medical, and psychological help must be given to the alcoholic or death will occur. By this time, he may have severe liver damage and possible brain tissue damage.

In this or the previous stage he or she is most likely to experience the "DT's," or delirium tremens. This reaction is characterized by delirium, muscle tremor, confusion, and hallucinations or delusions (mainly visual, such as moving animals, but tactile hallucinations may occur that cause alcoholics to feel that small animals or bugs are crawling on their skin). DT's do not generally occur until the alcoholic has been in the last two phases of alcoholism for several years, and at the onset of DT's the alcoholic may hallucinate only occasionally, but the symptoms gradually increase in duration and intensity. The psychotic episode lasts from two days to two weeks, frequently terminating in a long, deep sleep. In about 10% of the cases death occurs, mainly due to pneumonia, complete renal shutdown, or cardiac arrest [17].

During any one of these phases, alcoholics may change their drinking pattern to one of partial or complete abstinence. It is believed that once chronic drinkers can no longer control their drinking, that is, can no longer stop at one or two drinks, they cannot return to a social drinking status, but must become totally abstinent. Alcoholics Anonymous calls for this complete abstinence and has been the most effective agency in the nation in helping alcoholics recover.

In this modern day of psychology and social awareness, it is quite obvious that treating alcoholics is not merely a medical problem. Alcoholism is a social disease, calling for the help of the social psychologist in rehabilitating the alcoholic.

ITEM 19:   Personality disturbance is a basic reason for the development of alcoholism.

Answer

Many authorities on alcoholism and its treatment indicate that, in general, only individuals with serious personality maladjustments become chronic alcoholics [3].

'arious studies on alcoholism have shown that alcoholics tend to be insecure, nxious, and oversensitive, and dissatisfied with themselves and their lives as they re leading them [7]. Without alcohol they feel inferior to others and find it difficult o socialize or feel at ease in most social situations [20].

Although personality maladjustment may be a basic characteristic of the alco-iolic, it is not the only hypothesized "cause" of alcoholism. A second proposal or heory is that alcoholism is the result of a biochemical defect, a lack of certain body hemicals, perhaps enzymes or hormones [11, 13]. This theory contends that be-ause of a genetic deficiency, certain enzyme systems are not produced in the body. This creates a biological state or balance that can be maintained only by the intake »f alcohol. Animal studies have been conducted that show that rats with a vitamin B_1 deficiency prefer a mixture of water and alcohol to water alone [19]. Alcoholics Anonymous may prefer this theory, since members of this group have been known o report that they have an "allergy" to alcohol—something physical has caused heir alcoholism reaction [12].

The third basic causative factor that has been proposed is that of social dis-orientation [4, 20]. Bales [2] suggests that the rate of alcoholism in a society lepends on the following factors:

1. The degree to which the society brings about a need for escape—how much he society causes inner tensions in its members. In search of society-set goals, indi-viduals may become so pressured that they must find an escape, and alcohol be-omes that escape [5].

2. The kind of attitudes toward drinking that the society engenders in its members. Because drinking has become a sign of being "grown-up" and is often regarded as he socially acceptable thing to do, typical American youth may actually be pres-ured into drinking alcohol. Adult drinkers set the trend for the younger members of ociety. When alcohol is used in the home without fanfare or is used for religious purposes, it is less likely that members of those homes will use alcohol unwisely [4].

3. The number of suitable substitute means of satisfaction that the society pro-vides. When a society offers a variety of suitable means for its members to occupy heir thoughts and release tensions, self-destructive habits such as chronic drinking or any other drug habit will be less prevalent than in societies offering no socially acceptable escapes. For instance, some societies may offer religion as a form of escape. Also, a habit as simple as eating food may become a substitute escape mechanism.

In summary, it is only possible to state that there is no *one* cause of alcoholism, out probably a combination of several factors—psychological, social, and physio-ogical (see Fig. 3.3).

TEM 20: There is no cure for alcoholism.

Answer

t is generally agreed that once a person falls into the "true addiction" phase of lcoholism, he or she is thereafter considered an alcoholic. Many recovered alco-

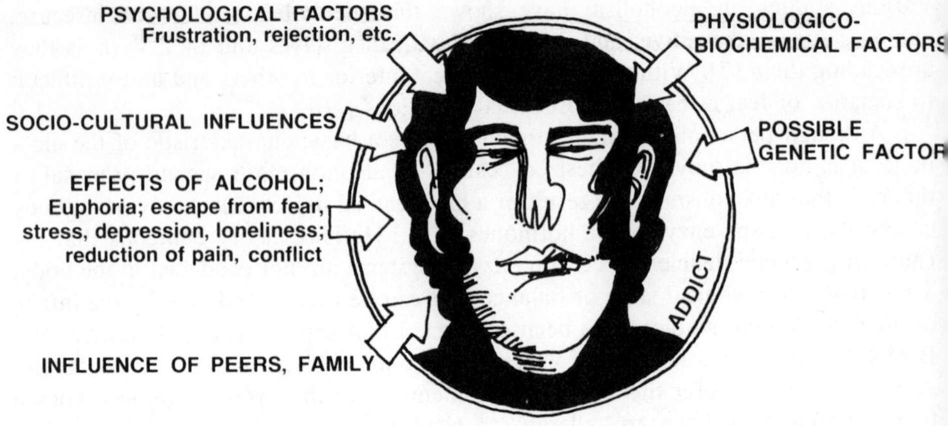

PSYCHOLOGICAL FACTORS
Frustration, rejection, etc.

PHYSIOLOGICO-
BIOCHEMICAL FACTORS

SOCIO-CULTURAL INFLUENCES

POSSIBLE
GENETIC FACTOR

EFFECTS OF ALCOHOL;
Euphoria; escape from fear,
stress, depression, loneliness;
reduction of pain, conflict

ADDICT

INFLUENCE OF PEERS, FAMILY

Fig. 3.3 Causative factors in alcoholism.

holics may prefer to call themselves "nonpracticing" alcoholics, but do admit that they are still alcoholics.

Alcoholics Anonymous members readily admit that they are alcoholics, and appear proud to say it because to them it means that they know their disease and have done something about it.

Even though there is no known "cure" for alcoholism, treatment is available to alcoholics at any stage in their drinking career. However, most alcoholics make their appearance in the hospital wards and rehabilitation groups only after their drinking has reached a critical point.

Upon presentation for medical service, the alcoholic is given vitamin (especially vitamin B) shots, is put on a special diet, and goes through a "drying out" period during which he or she is watched very closely for symptoms of withdrawal and is given medication (usually tranquilizers) to allay a number of withdrawal symptoms. After this initial medical phase has removed the alcoholic from imminent physical danger, social and psychological rehabilitation must follow in order to keep the alcoholic from lapsing back into alcohol use.

There are as many reasons for drinking as there are drinkers and, accordingly, there are nearly as many different kinds of alcoholic treatment programs as there are alcoholics. Careful scrutiny of the literally thousands of programs will show that each is an adaptation of the few basic techniques that are discussed below.

Psychotherapy forms the basis for many programs operating on the assumption that excessive drinking is (1) a psychoneurotic behavior that offers escape from grief, pain, anger, and guilt; (2) a release from anxiety, hostility, or feelings of inferiority; or (3) a means of dealing with unresolved feelings of sexual inadequacy, social weakness, or general rejection.

In addition to the use of psychotherapy, treatment modalities may involve the use of behavior modification. Aversion therapy is an example of how behavior modification is used in the treatment of alcoholism [8]. It involves teaching deeply relaxed patients to visualize themselves drinking, becoming sick, and eventually omiting, or to first visualize distasteful scenes, then think of drinking. Later they re taught to visualize feelings of well-being and associate these with being sober. Typnosis may be used, especially with subjects who find drinking euphoric and leasurable. In some cases effective use has been made of posthypnotic suggestions uch as, "I will never drink another drop in any form, for alcohol is meaningless and am indifferent to it and to people who use it." Electrotherapy is also used as a conitioning device in aversion therapy. Techniques vary, but one common practice is o attach electrodes to the fingers or to the ear of the subject. Then, in a barroom etting, the patient is allowed to drink at will, but receives shocks when he or she oes so; the shocks continue until the drink is rejected.

A more popular reeducation program involving aversion therapy is conducted rith the help of the drug Antabuse (disulfiram). This drug interferes with the netabolism of alcohol; after the alcohol is converted to acetaldehyde, further breakown is blocked. The toxic acetaldehyde causes flushed face, headache, increased eart rate, heart palpitations, nausea, vomiting, and breathing difficulty. When used treatment, the alcoholic knows that he will become ill if he ingests alcohol. It is a sense a chemical conscience for the alcoholic.

Another drug occasionally used in the treatment of alcoholism (not in aversion nerapy) is LSD. The therapeutic actions are in the form of breaking down defenses nd allowing the alcoholic to relive traumatic experiences so that the anxiety associ-ted with them might be reduced. In addition, a transcendental occurrence can pro-ide a powerful emotional experience that may give the patient the feeling of change nrough the gaining of new insights into feelings and behavior.

The idea of gaining power and control over one's self is an ego-building experi-nce which helps rebuild self-concept. Biofeedback instrumentation has been used this manner as patients are taught to control brain waves (alpha, beta, theta tates) at will, reduce muscle tension, or voluntarily change the temperature of a articular body site. This not only aids in reducing anxiety and tension, but also ives the feeling of self-control over behavior that has been found to carry over into nose situations that heretofore led to drinking.

Exercise programs have also been successful in the treatment of alcoholism. As n alcoholic, the individual develops poor health habits, is out of touch with his r her body, and forgets what it is like to feel good physically. Exercise increases fit-ess, develops self-confidence, and reduces tension and anxiety. The importance of educing tension and anxiety cannot be overemphasized—it is the reason that most rograms use tranquilizing drugs in some part of their treatment regimen.

All psychological treatment is not on an individual basis: group therapy is also widely accepted treatment modality. It is usually less expensive and gives the atient a chance to develop abilities with which to deal effectively with social situa-ons. Psychodrama, role playing, and sensitivity group interaction break down de-ense mechanisms and allow patients to see themselves in a more positive light and o analyze their relationship to the rest of society, especially to their family. Family essions helping to reestablish communication and to analyze problems that caused rustration are worked out with the help of a therapist.

A larger group approach, Alcoholics Anonymous, is perhaps the most successful of all group treatment modalities. This organization's basic aim is to help alcoholics stop drinking. Through group discussions with others who have similar problems, the alcoholic can come to realize that his or her problem is not unique and that other individuals have met the challenge of alcoholism successfully. Alcoholics Anonymous offers group identity, status, and prestige, qualities sorely lacking in the life of the alcoholic. With self-identity restored (or gained for the first time) the nonpracticing alcoholic is able to work toward regaining a normal life.

Since AA was founded in 1935 it has provided help for hundreds of thousands of people. The first step, that of admitting to be powerless over alcohol, is a difficult one and may come only after other forms of individual treatment. But once this is achieved, the alcoholic usually is able to refrain from taking the first drink, while each day of sobriety adds to his or her self-confidence. AA is a way of life for the nonpracticing alcoholic; a club or fraternitylike atmosphere develops and most social activities of AA members revolve around that group. Members become dedicated to helping others remain sober, which becomes a form of egotistic altruism. By helping others they help themselves.

In addition to the help given the alcoholic, AA offers aid in understanding the alcoholic mate or parent in their Alanon and Alateen groups. Here, nonalcoholic family members may learn about the disease of alcoholism and, more important, that the nonalcoholic is not responsible for the actions of the alcoholic. Guilt is an emotion common to family members of alcoholics, as they feel that they are the cause of the situations that drive the alcoholic to drink.

At the beginning of the chapter the staggering cost of alcoholism to society was mentioned. Millions are spent on rehabilitation, but this amount is miniscule when compared to what absenteeism, turnover, and accidents cost business and industry. For that reason a constantly increasing number of industries in the United States are now providing facilities for the early detection and treatment of alcoholism in their employees. Recent court decisions and shifts in public attitudes emphasizing the alcoholic disease concept, together with changing insurance company policy, have been largely responsible for this movement. While some segments of society have not responded, thus denying treatment-cost benefits provided for by health care programs, many insurance companies have recognized alcoholism under their mental health benefits. A major stumbling block is the usual insurance company provision that treatment be undertaken in a strictly medical setting in an accredited hospital (which usually offers very limited, expensive, and inefficient programs for the alcoholic). However, with the increasing development of data on treatment effectiveness, cost, licensing, and certification of facilities, insurance companies are expected to expand their coverage.

Business and industry interest is largely a matter of protecting dollars invested in employee training, and losses through absenteeism, production inefficiency, and accidents. The world's largest employer, the United States federal government, has led the way with the development of treatment programs, and grants to private industry for training key personnel in the Troubled Employee Program, a program emphasizing detection of employees who for whatever reason are not fulfilling their

b responsibilities. Foremen refer the employee to the personnel, medical, or coun-
ling unit of the company and diagnosis of the problem is made by qualified person-
el. A problem drinker can be referred to company or community programs and
an ever-increasing number of instances, the employee can be treated without los-
g his or her job.

EFERENCES

1. Adams, L. D., *The Common Sense Book of Drinking*. New York: David McKay, 1960.

2. Bales, R. F., "Cultural Difference in Rate of Alcoholism," in R. G. McCarthy, ed., *Drinking and Intoxication*, pp. 263–277. New York: Free Press, 1959.

3. Blane, H. T., *The Personality of the Alcoholic: Guises of Dependency*. New York: Harper & Row, 1968.

4. Chafetz, M. E., and H. W. Demone, Jr., *Alcoholism and Society*. New York: Oxford University Press, 1962.

5. Crosby, W. H., "Those Two Martinis Before Dinner Every Night," *Journal of the American Medical Association*, 231(5):509, 1975.

6. Davis, V. E., and M. J. Welsh, "Alcohol, Amines, and Alkaloids: A Possible Biochemical Basis for Alcohol Addiction," *Science*, 167:1005, 1970.

7. Dudley, D. L., *et al.*, "Heroin vs. Alcohol Addiction—Quantifiable Psychosocial Similarities and Differences," *Journal of Psychosomatic Research*, 18(5):327–335, 1974.

8. Elkins, R. L., "Aversion Therapy for Alcoholism," *International Journal of the Addictions*, 10(2):157–210, 1975.

9. Hayman, M., *Alcoholism: Mechanism and Management*. Springfield, Ill.: Charles C. Thomas, 1966.

0. Himwich, H. E., "The Metabolism and Pharmacology of Alcohol," in R. J. Catanzaro, ed., *Alcoholism*, pp. 26–38. Springfield, Ill.: Charles C. Thomas, 1968.

1. Hoff, C. E., "Pharmacologic and Metabolic Adjuncts," in R. J. Catanzaro, ed., *Alcoholism*, pp. 175–185. Springfield, Ill.: Charles C. Thomas, 1968.

2. Hore, B. D., "Craving for Alcohol," *British Journal of Addiction*, 69(2):137–140, 1974.

3. Jellinek, E. M., *The Disease Concept of Alcoholism*. Highland Park, N.J.: Hillhouse, 1968.

4. Jellinek, E. M., "Phases of Alcohol Addiction," *Quarterly Journal of Studies on Alcohol*, 13:672, 1952.

5. Kendis, J. B., "The Human Body and Alcohol," in D. J. Pittman, ed., *Alcoholism*, pp. 23–30. New York: Harper & Row, 1967.

6. Klatskin, G., "Effect of Alcohol on the Liver," *Reprint for Council on Foods and Nutrition of the AMA*, No. 36, November 1968.

17. Lieber, C. S., *et al.,* "Difference in Hepatic Metabolism of Long- and Medium-Cha Fatty Acids," *Journal of Clinical Investigation,* 46:1451–1460, 1967.

18. Lieber, C. S., and L. M. DeCarli, "An Experimental Model of Alcohol Feedi and Liver Injury in the Baboon," *Journal of Medical Primatology,* 3:153–163, 197

19. Mardones, R. J., "On the Relationship Between Deficiency of B Vitamins and A cohol Intake in Rats," *Quarterly Journal of Studies on Alcohol,* 12:563, 1951.

20. McCord, W., and J. McCord, *Origins of Alcoholism.* Palo Alto, Calif.: Stanfo University Press, 1960.

21. Skinner, H. A., *et al.,* "Alcoholic Personality Types," *Journal of Abnormal Ps chology,* 836:658–666, 1974.

22. United States Department of Health, Education, and Welfare, National Institutes Mental Health, *Alcohol and Health.* Washington, D.C.: U.S. Government Printi Office, 1974.

23. Westerfield, W. W., and M. P. Schulman, "Metabolism and Caloric Value of Alc hol," *Reprint for Council on Foods and Nutrition of the American Medical Ass ciation,* No. 33, August 1967.

SUGGESTED READING

Al-Anon Family Group, *Living With an Alcoholic.* New York: Al-Anon, 1965.

Bacon, M. K., *et al., Cross-Cultural Study of Drinking.* New Brunswick, N.J.: Rutge Center of Alcohol Studies, 1965.

Bacon, S. D., ed., *Driving and Drinking.* New Brunswick, N.J.: Rutgers Center of A cohol Studies, 1967.

Bihari, B., "Alcoholism in M.M.T.P. Patients," *National Conference on Methado Treatment Proceedings,* 1:288–295, 1973.

Block, Marvin A., *Alcoholism, Its Facets and Phases.* New York: John Day, 1965.

Brunn, Kettil, and Ragnar Hange, *Drinking Habits Among Northern Youth.* Ne Brunswick, N.J.: Rutgers Center of Alcohol Studies, 1963.

Cain, Arthur H., *Young People and Drinking.* New York: John Day, 1963.

Chafetz, Morris E., *Liquor: the Servant of Man.* Boston: Little, Brown, 1965.

Cooperative Commission on the Study of Alcoholism, *Alcohol Problems: a Report to th Nation.* New York: Oxford University Press, 1967.

Forney, Robert B., and Francis W. Highes, *Combined Effects of Alcohol and Othe Drugs.* Springfield, Ill.: Charles C. Thomas, 1968.

Fox, Ruth, *Alcoholism: Behavior Research, Therapeutic Approaches.* New York: Spe cer, 1967.

Garitano, W. W., *et al.,* "Concepts of Life Style in the Treatment of Alcoholism," *Inte national Journal of the Addictions,* 9(4):585–592, 1974.

Holloway, Elma, *Alcohol and Youth.* New York: Vantage Press, 1961.

Kent, P., *American Women and Alcohol.* New York: Holt, Rinehart, and Winston, 196 essel, Neil, and Harry Walton, *Alcoholism*. New York: Humanities Press, 1966.

insey, Barry A., *Female Alcoholic*. Springfield, Ill.: Charles C. Thomas, 1966.

evinson, D., "The Etiology of Skid Rows in the United States," *Social Psychiatry,* 0(1–2):25–33, 1974.

olli, Giorgio, *Social Drinking: How to Enjoy Drinking Without Being Hurt by it*. Cleve-nd: World, 1960.

olli, Giorgio, *et al., Alcohol in Italian Culture*. New Haven, Conn.: College and Uni-rsity Press, 1965.

addox, G. L., "Teenagers and Alcohol: Recent Research," *Annals of the New York cademy of Sciences,* 133:787, 1966.

addox, G. L., and Bevode C. McCall, *Drinking Among Teen-Agers*. New Brunswick, I.J.: Rutgers Center of Alcohol Studies, 1964.

aickel, Roger P., *Biochemical Factors in Alcoholism*. New York: Pergamon, 1967.

endelson, J. H., ed., *Alcoholism*. Boston: Little, Brown, 1965.

ullan, Hugh, and I. Sangiuliano, *Alcoholism: Group Psychotherapy and Rehabilita-on*. Springfield, Ill.: Charles C. Thomas, 1966.

arker, E. S., *et al.,* "Alcohol and the Disruption of Cognitive Processes," *Archives of eneral Psychiatry,* 31(6):824–828, 1974.

ittman, D. J., and C. W. Gordon, *Revolving Door*. New Haven, Conn.: College and niversity Press, 1965.

laut, T. F. A., *Alcohol Problems: a Report to the Nation by the Cooperative Commis-on on the Study of Alcoholism*. New York: Oxford University Press, 1967.

ollmer, Elizabeth, *Alcoholic Personalities*. New York: Exposition, 1965.

adoun, Roland, *et al., Drinking in French Culture*. New Brunswick, N.J.: Rutgers enter of Alcohol Studies, 1965.

hipp, T. J., *Helping the Alcoholic and his Family*. Englewood Cliffs, N.J.: Prentice-all, 1963.

nyder, C. R., *Alcohol and the Jews*. New Haven, Conn.: College and University Press, 965.

ahka, Viekko, *Alcoholic Personality*. New Brunswick, N.J.: Rutgers Center of Alcohol tudies, 1966.

odd, Frances, *Teaching about Alcohol*. New York: McGraw-Hill, 1964.

rice, H. M., *Alcoholism in America*. New York: McGraw-Hill, 1966.

nited States Department of Health, Education, and Welfare, *Alcohol Education: Con-rence Proceedings*. Washington, D.C.: U.S. Government Printing Office, 1966.

arner, H. S., *An Evolution in Understanding of the Problem of Alcohol: a History of ollege Idealism*. Boston: Christopher, 1966.

ylman, R., "Fatal Crashes Among Michigan Youth Following Reduction of Legal rinking Age," *Quarterly Journal of Studies on Alcohol,* 35:283–286, 1974.

ALCOHOL TERMINOLOGY

AA	Alcoholics Anonymous
Alkie	Alcoholic
Blackout	Temporary loss of memory from drinking alcohol
Bombed, Bombed out	Intoxicated
Booze	Alcoholic beverages
D & D	Drunk and disorderly (law enforcement term)
DT's	Delerium tremens, the alcohol withdrawal syndrome, characterized by nausea, vomiting, hallucinations, convulsions
DWI	Driving while intoxicated
FAC	Friday Afternoon Club, 5:00 Friday afternoon drinking group, popular on college campuses
Hard stuff	Whiskey, gin, rum, etc.
High	Intoxicated
John Barleycorn	Alcoholic beverages, usually referring to whiskey
Juiced up	Intoxicated
Revolving door	Pertaining to alcoholics continually returning to alcohol after making some rehabilitative effort
Shakes (the)	DT's, or the beginning stages of the DT's
Smashed	Intoxicated
Squiffed	Intoxicated
Suds	Beer

MARIJUANA: THE GREAT DEBATE

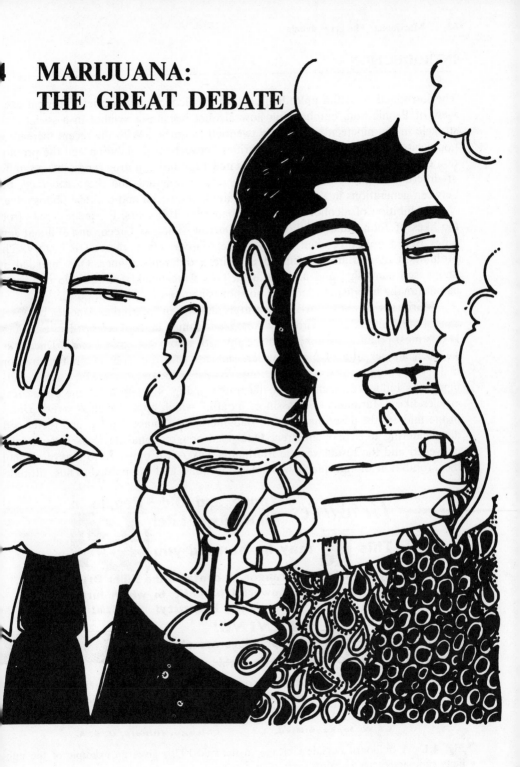

INTRODUCTION

The introduction to the preceding chapter on alcohol gave a brief historical over view of Prohibition, emphasizing how alcohol became a symbol in a social clas struggle in the nineteenth and early twentieth centuries. With the recent increase i popularity of marijuana, many similarities between its prohibition and the prohib tion of alcohol have been drawn. In this new prohibition a drug represents a symbc of differences not between the working class immigrant and the aristocracy, bu between generations in their life styles, values, and social and political philosophies

Prohibition of alcohol was hotly debated for 100 years. Eloquent debate fror the likes of John Stuart Mill, Clarence Darrow, Thomas Green, and William Jen nings Bryan finally resulted in popular legislative action; the rest is history. Th prohibition of marijuana occurred in quite a different manner. One man led a unopposed campaign and antimarijuana laws were quickly passed. No one reall cared, for the marijuana users had no spokesmen and no political power.

Marijuana has been used for centuries and was introduced in America by Mexi can laborers and later imported by American seamen in the southeast United States It was most popular among jazz musicians with whom it migrated north. During th 1930s headlines told of mass murder, suicides, and robberies committed by nor mally law-abiding citizens who were under the influence of the killer weed, mari juana. As billboards such as that illustrated in Fig. 4.1 appeared, the public read articles like "Marijuana—Assassin of Youth," which appeared in *Reader's Diges* in the mid-1930s, describing human slaughterhouses, mass murder, and reefer ped dlers catering to school children. One-sided congressional hearings were quickly convened and the result was the Marijuana Tax Act. Compared to that of alcohol the prohibition of marijuana was relatively quite and unopposed. Thus, attitudes

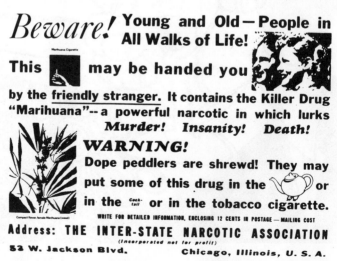

Fig. 4.1 A billboard outside Chicago in the mid-1930s gives an example of the pub- licity campaign waged against marijuana.

ɔward marijuana developed in this vein and little was heard on the subject until the ublicity surrounding the beatniks and hippies created the controversy that exists ɔday.

The great debate concerning marijuana initially centered on the physical harm of he substance. However, voluminous reports from disagreeing experts rendered this ssue practically unsolvable. Advocates of the liberalization of marijuana laws conɔnd that the use of marijuana is a private, moral decision and that any resulting ιarm accrues only to the user. They further feel that those who oppose its use are nterfering with essentially private conduct that is a basic freedom guaranteed by the Constitution. Defenders of the present restrictions insist that society has not only he right, but also the duty, to protect existing social order and to compel individuals ɔ abstain from behavior that impairs productivity and social responsibility. Howɔver, all arguments are not that rational. The easy-going, pleasure-seeking "hippie" ifestyle engendered fear of social disorder, lack of responsibility, and moral decay. Γhe lines were drawn and opinions hardened, while emotions replaced logic; thus, narijuana became the symbol of a disagreement between social and moral stability ιnd individual freedom.

As in the 1920s, the law enforcement apparatus was caught in the middle. Legal ɔnforcement of the prohibition of marijuana is virtually impossible. The costs are ɬtaggering, not only in monies for police, lawyers, and judges, but in the misery of ɔhose jailed for possession and use of what many regard as a harmless drug. Disrespect and fear of the legal establishment results from unequal enforcement of a ɦodgepodge of legal statutes.

It was clear that a uniform social policy was necessary; thus, in 1970 a Presidential Commission (The President's Commission on Marijuana and Drug Abuse [14]) was established to separate fiction from fact and to recommend a uniform policy that would not only reflect the attitudes of the majority, but also legally and morally provide for the freedoms of the individual. Officially, the Commission's findings did not result in legislative changes, but unofficially, enforcement policies seem to be moving in the directions outlined by the Commission. While recognizing the fact that several million citizens use marijuana without observable detriment to themselves or to society, the Commission's survey showed that dominant opinion still opposed marijuana use. The Commission could not recommend legalization of marijuana or even a position of neutrality toward it, since either position might signify society's approval of it and possible encouragement of its use. Instead, the Commission recommended a social policy of discouragement. It sought to increase the efforts of schools, churches, and families in implementation of the discouragement policy and to decrease the use of police powers for the regulation of what is essentially "private conduct."

The Commission sought to make a clear distinction between what constituted private conduct and what was public. The specific recommendation was that the possession of marijuana for personal use would no longer be a criminal offense, but marijuana possessed in public would remain contraband, subject to seizure. It further recommended that states adopt a uniform statutory scheme similar to the proposed federal laws, in which private possession would not be considered a criminal

offense, possession of small amounts in public would be punishable by a fine, an
sale would remain a serious offense with stringent penalties.

The Commission's distinction between possession and sale was both philosoph
cal and practical—practical because the supply system for marijuana, like all drug
is pyramidal. At the top are few people with a lot of marijuana, and at the botto
are many people with a little marijuana. It is more justified and feasible for la
enforcement agencies to direct their efforts toward the few at the top, the distribu
tors. Philosophically, this would be in accord with the purpose of the legal apparatu
—to regulate public behavior while not infringing upon activity conducted withi
the confines of one's own home.

One sign of change in public sentiment was evidenced by the fact that a grou
of Californians raised enough support to have included on the 1972 ballot a refer
endum that would decriminalize the use of marijuana. This was Proposition 19, th
California Marijuana Initiative, which operated on the premise that any society tha
values personal freedom and the right to privacy should use the criminal proces
sparingly, and only when necessary to control conduct that threatens the right o
the public in general. In the eyes of the supporters of Proposition 19 marijuana wa
not harmful and enforcement of the existing laws was costing not only the individua
user, but also the taxpayers by overburdening the legal system. Results of the surve
carried out by the President's Commission, indicating that the average America
was not ready to legalize or decriminalize the use of marijuana, were borne out i
California as Proposition 19 was soundly defeated. It seems likely that initiative
that now decriminalize possession of small amounts (1–1½ oz.) of marijuana i
Oregon, Alaska, Colorado, Maine, and California will reach the ballot in othe
states in the next few years, but the success or failure of such initiatives depends o
how each individual interprets the often-conflicting reports concerning marijuana

To help educate society and to make sure that lawmakers and politicians were
kept abreast of the latest scientific information the Pot lobby (the National Organization for the Reform of Marijuana, or NORML) was formed in 1970. This wa
a significant event, for it represented the first nationally organized movement to do
away with marijuana prohibition. NORML used a middle-class, pragmatic, time-
honored lobbying style to get legislators to accept the recommendation of the President's Commission, that of decriminalization of marijuana users (not legalization of
marijuana). They continually emphasized that while the scientists debate the question of the dangers of marijuana, thousands are being punished for using what might
be later found to be a relatively harmless drug.

The remainder of this chapter presents in summary form the facts about marijuana, especially those pertinent to the question of legalization.

CANNABIS

Nearly any student of drugs can supply the fact that marijuana is derived from the
flowers and the top leaves of the female *Cannabis sativa* plant, a weed of the hemp

amily which flourishes without the necessity of special cultivation. The resin, a ticky yellow substance, is produced by the plant as a protective shield against the elements; marijuana plants grown in hotter, sunnier climates produce more resin in order to protect themselves from the sun's heat. (These plants are the most highly sought because the marijuana produced from them will be stronger!) The active ingredient in marijuana is thought to be tetrahydrocannabinol, specifically, delta 9 tetrahydrocannabinol, with possible synergistic effects from other cannabidiols and cannabinols. The effects on humans are highly dependent on the dose administered.

There are a number of basic preparations of cannabis, the strength of each depending on the amount of active tetrahydrocannabinol (THC) that it contains. In the United States the weakest, and most widely used, preparation is derived from the tops of uncultivated flowering shoots and is simply called "marijuana" (or "grass," "weed," "MJ," and other nicknames *ad infinitum*). The word is said to be derived from the Portuguese *mariguango,* which means "intoxicant." Much of the marijuana used in the United States is grown here and it is of a very weak variety; it is usually olive-green in color. Jamaican and Colombian marijuana is dark brown, Panama Red is a claylike red, and Acapulco Gold is dull yellow in color. All of these foreign types are stronger than the marijuana grown in the United States.

The cannabis used in the preparation of *bhang* in India is of similar potency to American marijuana and appears to be widely used there as a mild intoxicant with no great health or social hazard [3]. For a cannabis product of greater potency than *bhang,* the small leaves and resinous material are treated in such a manner that one solid mass is formed. This preparation is called *ganja* by the Indians. The most potent source of THC is the pure resin, which is carefully removed from the leaves of the plant. This gummy substance is called *charas* in India, but Americans are more likely to know it as hashish. Its potency is five to ten times that of marijuana, depending on growing conditions and how it is used [16]. The resin hardens into a brown lump, a darker color signifying increased potency. Reports vary, but hashish usually has between 5 and 20% THC. Forms of liquid hashish, called hash oil, may have between 20 and 70% THC.

Table 4.1 shows the cannabis potency continuum. Note that marijuana and *bhang* are of similar potency and that hashish and *charas* are merely different terms for the same substance.

In the Western world cannabis is usually smoked and in this form is considered more potent than when taken orally in drinks or food preparations [16], as is the

TABLE 4.1
Potency continuum of American and Indian cannabis preparations

	Low potency (0–1% THC)	Medium potency (0–5% THC)	High potency (5–20% THC)	Highest potency (20–70% THC)
United States	Domestic marijuana	Foreign marijuana	Hashish	Hash oil
India	*Bhang*	*Ganja*	*Charas*	

practice in Eastern countries. Smoking allows more control over the use of cannabis, because the effects can be felt much more rapidly and intake altered accordingly. Ingestion effects last longer, but nausea and vomiting may occur as an aftermath.

Partly because of the underlying compulsion of man to classify and identify, marijuana was tossed into the "narcotic" classification before its nature was known and it now appears to be a prisoner of this legislation classification. Although most people now concede that marijuana is not a narcotic, there is still considerable controversy over the classification of cannabis preparations, because their effects are highly dependent on dose. However, since marijuana is of the lowest potency among cannabis preparations, it must be considered to be a sedative-hypnotic, much like alcohol [3, 8, 11, 16]. There are those who prefer to advertise marijuana as being a psychedelic or hallucinatory substance, but they are most likely speaking of a stronger THC preparation than the "common garden variety" American marijuana.

PHYSICAL EFFECTS

One of the basic arguments against the use or legalization of marijuana is that since there is so little scientific evidence concerning its effects, we should treat it like any medical drug—before it can be used legally, it must be studied until it is proved harmless to humans. Although there are many biochemical aspects of marijuana that are yet to be uncovered, the stockpile of known physiological effects is growing.

The headlines shown here indicate the contradictory nature of reports appearing in newspapers, magazines, and scientific journals—the sources upon which the public relies for information regarding the effects of marijuana. Most articles represent the results of one study, most often valid in itself, but usually subject to certain limitations. The best information emanates from reports of many reproducible studies using similar variables.

Animal studies have given evidence that marijuana does not appreciably affect overt behavior or simple learning skills in rats, has a tranquilizing effect on aggressive mice, and causes a sleepy, dreamlike state (much like the later stage of the human high) in dogs. It has been found that an overdose will kill a cat (3 grams of *charas,* 8 grams of *ganja,* or 10 grams of *bhang,* each of these doses being grams per

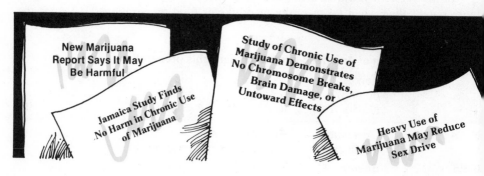

New Marijuana Report Says It May Be Harmful

Jamaica Study Finds No Harm in Chronic Use of Marijuana

Study of Chronic Use of Marijuana Demonstrates No Chromosome Breaks, Brain Damage, or Untoward Effects

Heavy Use of Marijuana May Reduce Sex Drive

kilogram of body weight [4]). Dogs have also been administered high doses and death has occurred from respiratory failure [11]. There are no known overdose cases in man that resulted in death.

Experimental studies on humans have substantiated animal studies showing nausea, diarrhea, vomiting, and failure of muscular coordination after use of marijuana, especially after an oral dose of the substance [3, 10, 16, 18].

It appears that reaction time to complex stimuli, steadiness of hand and body, visual and time perception, and intelligence test scores are adversely affected by marijuana [10]. More recent tests showed altered time sense, decreased auditory discrimination, difficulty in concentration, and impairment of ability in some psychometric tests, especially those related to the manipulation of numbers [5].

In the classic study done by Weil et al. [18], it was found that marijuana experiences and reactions depended on whether or not the user was familiar with marijuana at the time. "Naive" subjects did not experience the same kind of "high" that chronic marijuana users did, and their subsequent test performance scores suffered more from the marijuana experience than did the scores of those who knew the marijuana "high" from previous experience. Weil's group found that marijuana increases heart rate moderately and causes reddening of the conjunctivae (one of the surest signs of marijuana use), but does not produce any change in blood sugar level, in pupil size, or in respiratory rate.

Among the more important acute effects of marijuana are those associated with driving performance. Since marijuana produces effects similar to those caused by alcohol intoxication, attention is impaired, braking time is lengthened, and a total of more driving errors occur both in judgment and performance when driving under the influence of either of these two drugs. It has also been shown that glare recovery time (after driving into headlights at night, for example) is lengthened in marijuana-influenced drivers.

Although some recent studies on chronic high-dose marijuana use found typical withdrawal symptoms after abrupt withdrawal of the drug, most authorities still agree that physical dependence does not develop. Dose-dependent tolerance does seem to develop [15], but authorities are not sure whether this tolerance is pharmacological or due to learning factors (i.e., learning to perform more normally during the altered state). Thus, when considering the average use patterns of Americans, tolerance to marijuana is not of major consequence.

Investigation into the long-term or chronic effects of marijuana have produced inconclusive results of which one can only say that they are significant enough to study further. Preliminary findings of marijuana-related impairment of the immune response [13] could be significant in the etiology of infectious disease. Another area of investigation that bears study is the marijuana-related reduction in testosterone level and sperm count [7], resulting in impotence and decreased fertility. Again, these are only preliminary findings. Chromosome abnormalities have been found to be associated with marijuana use but no significant cytogenic effects have been accepted. Any drug may produce teratogenic effects and all unprescribed drugs should be avoided during pregnancy [17].

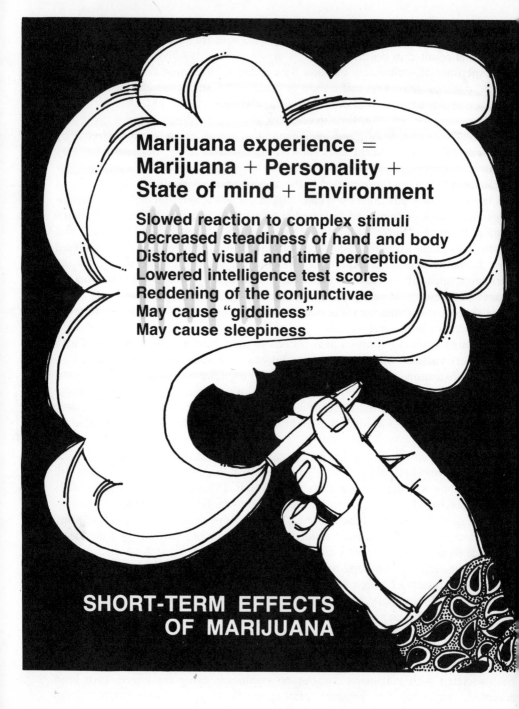

**Marijuana experience =
Marijuana + Personality +
State of mind + Environment**

Slowed reaction to complex stimuli
Decreased steadiness of hand and body
Distorted visual and time perception
Lowered intelligence test scores
Reddening of the conjunctivae
May cause "giddiness"
May cause sleepiness

**SHORT-TERM EFFECTS
OF MARIJUANA**

The American Medical Association says: "The inhaled [marijuana] smoke is irritating, and long continued exposure to it induces chronic respiratory disorders" [1]. Although this statement is not documented with a specific study, one could intuitively suggest this argument from what we know about tobacco smoking and respiratory complications. It is interesting that some of the harshness and throat irritation caused by marijuana is due to the cola used as a cohesive agent by those who illegally package Mexican marijuana for shipment.

The phenomenon of "flashbacks" is well known in the literature on drug abuse, but is usually associated with LSD or other hallucinogenic experiences. Some investigators have reported such occurrences, but Smith [16] has found no such occurrences in the large marijuana-using population of the Haight-Ashbury community in San Francisco, and seriously doubts other reports of such incidents. Marijuana (as well as alcohol, restricted movement, and psychedelics) can, and does, trigger "flashbacks" to a previous LSD experience, and this may be the confusing factor that has led to the belief in the existence of marijuana "flashbacks."

In summary, it can be said that, to date, purely *physical* effects of marijuana have not been found to be permanently damaging, except for the possibility of respiratory tract irritation (not fully documented at this time). This statement in itself may give all the information that some people wish to know, but the fact that we now know of no permanent physical damage caused by smoking marijuana is no guarantee that there are no such hazards. More important, long-term physical effects on the individual are not our only concern in this issue. Any time a depressant drug is taken by an individual who assumes responsibility for others' safety (as in driving a car), full responsibility cannot be taken because the drug-depressed state entails the loss of a number of essential qualities that enable a person to make rational decisions. In the case of marijuana depression, the subject's inhibitions, body control, visual and time perception, braking time, and glare recovery are affected to a certain extent, depending on the individual, the environment, and the quality and quantity of the marijuana. In this indirect manner, then, long-term physical damage could result from marijuana use.

Again, a word of caution to those who continually follow marijuana research as it is printed: Study the document for the number of experimental and control subjects used, the potency of the substance in terms of THC per kilogram of body weight used, mode of administration, setting, and other aspects of valid experimental research. Isbell [6] found that doses as small as 120 *micro*grams per kilogram body weight of synthetic THC administered orally or 50 micrograms per kg taken by smoking brought about effects similar to those that occurred after smoking a marijuana cigarette. Also, in the study done by Weil *et al.* [18] the "high" dose administered was around 18 milligrams per subject. According to Hollister [5], the average marijuana cigarette contains about 500 milligrams of marijuana with one percent THC content. With a 50% delivery, the smoker would take in 2.5 milligrams of THC. The dosage used in many experimental situations would be closer to that obtained from a number of marijuana cigarettes of high THC content or from hashish.

PSYCHOSOCIAL EFFECTS

From the surveys showing incidence of marijuana use on college campuses it should be evident that marijuana has little or no effect on intelligence. This has been borne out by controlled laboratory experiments. Numerous investigators have failed to find any significant differences in motivation factors or class standing when comparing marijuana users with nonusers. The psychological tests currently available for use cannot detect significant differences between moderate users and nonusers, but it has been shown that chronic marijuana use seems to correlate with manifest psychopathology. A revealing study by Mirin *et al.* [12] identified some of the personality differences between casual (1 to 4 times per month) and heavy (20 to 30 times per month) marijuana users. They found the abuser of marijuana to be psychologically similar to abusers of other drugs. The heavy marijuana user was a multiple drug user. He exhibited some degree of psychological dependence, manifested by anxiety when supply was low, and a self-perceived inability to relate to the world in general when not high. Heavy users were judged to have a poorer work adjustment and a self-reported inability to master new problems. Heavy users expressed a poor heterosexual adjustment and were judged to be more hostile toward society, more depressed, and to have more anxieties than casual users. The average casual user was not unlike the average nonuser in the above-mentioned categories.

It is highly doubtful that it is the marijuana that causes the psychological problem; there must first be a personality that needs a chemical escape (the same is true for alcohol or any other drug). Smith [16] proposes that the proportion of "potheads" in the total population of marijuana users parallels that of alcoholics in the population of alcohol users. We know that not all those who drink alcohol will become alcoholics; hence, we should take heart that not all marijuana smokers will become hopelessly dependent upon it. However, it is clear that the United States, having six to seven million alcoholics, does not also wish to have six to seven million marijuana dependents, a conceivable consequence of unrestricted use of marijuana.

Marijuana use does go against the mores and customs of the United States, and reports of use in other countries do not justify its use in the United States. However, these foreign reports do show that some people can use it and still function adequately in their society. Chopra and Chopra [2], reporting on use in India, reveal that when it is consumed legally, there are few complications and anxieties caused by fear of the law; there is, however, simple relief from the hardships imposed by poverty. Their often quoted statement adequately sums up possible motivations for use in India:

> A common practice amongst laborers engaged in building or excavation work is to have a few pulls on a ganja pipe, or to drink a glass of bhang towards the evening. This produces a sense of well-being, relieves fatigue, stimulates the appetite, and induces a feeling of mild stimulation, which enables the worker to bear more cheerfully the strain and perhaps the monotony of the daily routine of life. [2]

They point out that marijuana is a mild intoxicant that tends to suppress rather than excite aggressive or criminal behavior. Marijuana intoxication normally induces a state of lethargy rather than excitement, and while it may release inhibitions it will not make a criminal of a noncriminal or vice versa.

Marijuana psychosis

A commonly debated point concerning marijuana is that of marijuana-induced psychosis. The forces that precipitate a "psychotic reaction" are as varied as the individuals experiencing them. Psychosis may be triggered by tension, tragedy, stress from a multitude of causes, or possibly marijuana; but statistics indicate that marijuana psychosis is very rare. In marijuana-smoking populations no more psychosis has been observed than in a nonusing population. In 1967 San Francisco General Hospital treated more than 5000 cases of acute drug intoxication, yet no marijuana psychoses were seen. Haight-Ashbury Clinic has seen no marijuana psychosis in 30,000 patients, of whom 95% were marijuana users. Theoretically, marijuana or any other mind-altering chemical has the potential of bringing out symptoms that can be called "psychotic reactions" in a psychotic individual, but few have been reported to date [16].

The marijuana-using population

The marijuana-using population changed a good deal between 1940 and 1970; however, public attitude toward users did not, for the using group remained a distinct subculture, identifiable by sloppy dress, long hair, and liberal political views. These characteristics were included in the often-studied, overpublicized "marijuana personality," a personality lacking motivation, discipline, and values. Studies designed to discover the relationship between marijuana use and personality deviation showed that users tended to be more alienated from established society, but it could not be concluded whether alienation was the cause of marijuana use or an effect of society's labeling marijuana users as deviant for choosing that drug. Actually, it was a combination of the two plus a third that is not time-linked with the counterculture; that is, since marijuana use magnifies and intensifies feelings of altered reality, the relationship between self and reality is also altered. As reality is dictated by the established morality- and value-makers, an altered sense of reality leads to alienation. Concomitants of the drug state are altered time sense, and changes in perception, sensory awareness, memory, emotion, and moods. The more the drug is used, the more reality is altered, creating subtle changes in the user's concept of reality and self. Engaging in everyday activities such as eating or listening to music become new experiences because they are seen and felt differently. Instead of automatically performing a function without thinking, the user finds that he or she is intensively scrutinizing a given situation, as if suddenly turning and seeing the Grand Canyon for the first time—one stops and studies it, and ponders its wonder and significance. The activity itself is pleasurable and an end in itself—something to be experienced, not used. How one feels is more important than what one does. Thus, many chronic marijuana users in the counterculture developed concepts of self and reality that demanded more pleasure from each situation, and happiness came to be defined as immediate pleasure with little reverence of delayed gratification and the meeting of long-term needs.

The need to belong and to support the definition of reality acceptable to self and significant others led to the subsequent development of a subculture in which drugs, especially marijuana, were not only a symbol, but a balm to be used when the real world conflicted with a drug-induced reality.

Since the counterculture movement of the 1960s, the marijuana-using population has become largely indefinable with no one group cornering the market. It has been shown that male users outnumber female users, and that female use patterns tend to follow those of the girl's close male companions. Frequently, girls are first exposed to marijuana on dates or at parties; thus it follows that those more socially active are more likely to use marijuana. Premarital sexual intercourse and independent residence at college are also positively related to marijuana use, possibly showing a striving toward independence and openness to new experiences. Marijuana use seems to decrease when students leave college, which reflects separation from the student drug-using subculture, entrance into a larger, less tolerant society, a commitment to nonstudent rules, and increased job and family responsibilities. Change in drug use may also reflect increased maturity in the sense of accepting reality as seen by American society in general, and of finding one's self or place in society, reflecting less social alienation and an increase in independence or self-actualization. It might also be the final realization that happiness is not necessarily synonymous with pleasure and that the humanistic psychologist's view of happiness and fulfillment can be better attained by active, rather than passive, activities.

Abraham Maslow [9] characterized the drug experience as a temporary pleasure device, totally unreal, and thus unrelated to ongoing life. Fleeting glimpses into the self tempt one to go back for a better look and a better feeling. Overemphasis on the "feeling" world of subjective experiences may lead one to withdraw in order to search for triggers of such experiences, resulting in self-absorption and selfishness which diminish motivation to participate in the search for what Maslow terms growth experiences. These are experiences for which the person feels responsible. They are active and creative and are used as stepping stones toward additional growth, activities that meet long-term, psychological needs such as self-respect, self-esteem, and self-love. Often directed outward to one's fellow man, they overcome one's feeling of separateness and fulfill the need to belong.

Any of the surveys on motivation for marijuana use will show that curiosity, activity with friends, relaxation, and pleasure are the most often cited reasons for use. It is understandably difficult for respondents of these surveys to admit to such negative motivations as being pressured by peers, or needing marijuana as a coping device to escape from unpleasant situations. In the final analysis, initial experimentation is the result of curiosity and peer activity, but there are those chronic, heavy users who have chosen marijuana as their particular chemical escape. The reasons for use of the vast majority in the middle run the gamut from an interest in pleasurable sights, sounds, and feelings to a desire to soften the harshness of the real world. It is difficult to detect the difference between the seeking of pleasurable activity when bored, and quasi-pathological escapism. Of course, this may all be academic, for users may not contemplate their motivations; they simply seek that which satisfies them, in this case the effects of the drug. To a few marijuana offers glimpses of self-transcendence and insights into self, but little is learned from drugged experiences, for the altered state of consciousness does not communicate well with remembering, processing, learning, "I-Normal" consciousness. Thus, marijuana is not usually a growth activity or a means activity, but an end in itself.

REFERENCES

1. American Medical Association, "Dependence on Cannabis (Marihuana)," *Journal of the American Medical Association*," 201:368–371, 1967.

2. Chopra, R. N., and G. S. Chopra, "The Present Position of Hemp-Drug Addiction in India," *Bulletin on Narcotics*, 9:21–33, 1957.

3. Fort, J., "Has the World Gone to Pot?" *Journal of Psychedelic Drugs* (Haight-Ashbury Medical Clinic, San Francisco), 2(1), 1968.

4. Grinspoon, L., "Marihuana," *Scientific American*, 221:18–25, 1969.

5. Hollister, L. H., "Marihuana in Man: Three Years Later," *Science*, 172:21–29, 1971.

6. Isbell, H., *et al.*, "Effects of Δ^9-THC in Man," *Psychopharmacologia*, 11:184–188, 1967.

7. Kolodny, R. C., *et al.*, "Depression of Plasma Testosterone Levels After Chronic Intensive Marijuana Use," *New England Journal of Medicine*, 290:872–874, 1974.

8. Kubena, R. K., and H. Barry, "Interactions of 1-Tetrahydrocannabinol with Barbiturates and Methamphetamine," *Journal of Pharmacology and Experimental Therapeutics*, 173:94–100, 1970.

9. Maslow, A. H., *Motivation and Personality*. New York: Harper, 1954.

10. Mayor's Committee on Marihuana, *The Marihuana Problem in the City of New York*. New York, 1944.

11. Meyers, F. H., "Pharmacological Effects of Marijuana," *Journal of Psychedelic Drugs* (Haight-Ashbury Medical Clinic, San Francisco), 2(1), 1968.

12. Mirin, S. M., *et al.*, "Casual Versus Heavy Use of Marijuana: a Redefinition of the Marijuana Problem," *American Journal of Psychiatry*, 127(9):54–60, 1971.

13. Nahas, J., *et al.*, "Inhibition of Cellular Mediated Immunity in Marihuana Smokers," *Science*, 183:419, 1974.

14. National Commission on Marijuana and Drug Abuse, "Marijuana: A Signal of Misunderstanding," Washington, D.C.: U.S. Government Printing Office, 1972.

15. Perez-Reyes, M., *et al.*, "Long Term Use of Marihuana and the Development of Tolerance or Sensitivity to Delta-9-tetrahydrocannabinol," *Archives of General Psychiatry*, 31:89–91, 1974.

16. Smith, D. E., "Acute and Chronic Toxicity of Marijuana," *Journal of Psychedelic Drugs* (Haight-Ashbury Medical Clinic, San Francisco), 2(1), 1968.

17. United States Department of Health, Education, and Welfare, *Marijuana and Health* Washington, D.C.: U.S. Government Printing Office, 1974.
18. Weil, A. T., N. E. Zinberg, and J. M. Nelson, "Clinical and Psychological Effects o Marihuana in Man," *Science,* 162:1234–1242, 1969.

SUGGESTED READING

AMA Council on Mental Health, "Dependence on Cannabis (Marijuana)," *Journal o the American Medical Association,* 201:368–371, 1967.

AMA Council on Mental Health, "Marijuana and Society," *Journal of the America Medical Association,* 204:1181–1182, 1968.

Andrews, G., and S. Vinkenoog, eds., *The Book of Grass: an Anthology of Indian Hemp* New York: Grove Press, 1967.

Ball, John C., "Marihuana Smoking and the Onset of Heroin Use," *British Journal o Criminology,* 7:408–413, 1967.

Bloomquist, E. R., *Marijuana.* New York: Glencoe, 1971.

Bloomquist, E. R., "Marihuana: Social Benefit or Social Detriment?" *California Med cine,* 106:346, 1967.

Bonnie, R. J., and C. H. Whitebread II, *The Marihuana Conviction; A History of Mari huana Prohibition in the United States.* Charlottesville: University Press of Virginia 1974.

Bouquet, R. S., "Cannabis," *Bulletin on Narcotics,* 2:14–30, 1950.

Brill, N. O., *et al.,* "Marijuana Use and Psychosocial Adaptation," *Archives of Genera Psychiatry,* 31(5):713–719, 1974.

Chopra, R. N., "Cannabis Sativa in Relation to Mental Diseases and Crime in India," *Indian Journal of Medicine,* January 1942.

CIBA Foundation Study Group No. 21. *Hashish: Its Chemistry and Pharmacology* Boston: Little, Brown, 1965.

Clark, S. C., "Marijuana and the Cardiovascular System," *Pharmacology, Biochemistry and Behavior,* 3(2):299–306, 1975.

Coles, Robert, *The Grass Pipe.* Boston: Little, Brown, 1969.

Culver, C. M., *et al.,* "Neuropsychological Assessment of Undergraduate Marijuana and LSD Users," *Archives of General Psychiatry,* 31(5):707–711, 1974.

Eells, Kenneth, "Marihuana and LSD, a Survey of One College Campus," *Journal of Counseling Psychology,* 15:459–467, 1968.

Eells, K. W. *Pot: Medical and Psychological Aspects of Marihuana.* Pasadena: California Institute of Technology, 1968.

Ewing, J. A., "Students, Sex, and Marijuana," *Medical Aspects of Human Sexuality,* 7:101–117, 1972.

Fisher, G., "Milieu of Marijuana Use," *International Journal of Social Psychiatry,* 20(1–2):45–55, 1974.

Fort, Joel, *The Pleasure Seekers: the Drug Crisis, Youth, and Society.* Indianapolis: Bobbs-Merrill, 1969.

Geber, W. F., and L. C. Schram, "Effect of Marihuana Extraction on Fetal Hamsters and Rabbits," *Toxicology and Applied Pharmacology,* 14:276–282, 1969.

Goodes, Erich, ed., *Marihuana.* New York: Atherton, 1969.

Grinspoon, Lester, *Marijuana Reconsidered.* Cambridge, Mass.: Harvard University Press, 1971.

Grupp, Stanley E., "Observations on Experienced and Exclusive Marihuana Smokers," *Journal of Drug Issues,* 2:32–36, 1972.

Halikas, J. A., *et al.,* "Pattern of Marihuana Use: a Survey of One Hundred Regular Users," *Comprehensive Psychiatry,* 13:161–163, 1972.

Harmon, J. W., *et al.,* "Marijuana-Induced Gynocomastia," *Surgical Forum,* 25:423–425, 1974.

Hodapp, A. E., *Marihuana: a Review of the Literature for Analytical Chemists.* U.S. Customs Laboratory, New Orleans, 1959.

Hollister, L. L., *et al.,* "Comparison of Tetrahydrocannabinol and Synhexyl in Man," *Clinical Pharmacology Therapeutics,* 9:783–791, 1968.

Johnson, R. D., "Why So Many Teenagers Fall for Marihuana," *Parents' Magazine,* 64:58, 1969.

Kaplan, John, *Marijuana: the New Prohibition.* New York: World Press, 1970.

Kaufman, Joshua, "Runaways, Hippies and Marihuana," *American Journal of Psychiatry,* 126:163–166, 1969.

Keeler, M. H., "Adverse Reaction to Marihuana," *American Journal of Psychiatry,* 124:674–677, 1967.

King, A. B., "Effect of Intravenous Injection of Marihuana," *Journal of the American Medical Association,* 210:724–725, 1969.

Lorentz, R. J., "Levels of Dogmatism and Attitudes toward Marijuana," *Psychological Reports,* 30:75–78, February 1972.

Manhiemer, D. I., *et al.,* "Marihuana Use Among Urban Adults," *Science,* 166:1544–1545, 1969.

McGlothlin, W. H., "Toward a Rational View of Marihuana," in J. L. Simmons, ed., *Marihuana, Myths and Realities.* New York: Brandon House, 1968.

McNally, L. R., "Parents' Guide to Marijuana," Sunnyvale, Calif.: Western Electric Manufacturing and Supply Unit of the Bell System, 1968.

Milman, Doris H., "The Role of Marihuana in Patterns of Drug Abuse by Adolescents," *Journal of Pediatrics,* 74:288–290, 1969.

Orcutt, J. D., and D. A. Biggs, "Recreational Effects of Marijuana and Alcohol," *International Journal of the Addictions,* 10(2):229–240, 1975.

Pet, D. D., and J. C. Ball, "Marihuana Smoking in the United States," *Federal Probation,* 32:8–15, 1968.

Rosevear, John, *Pot: a Handbook of Marijuana.* New Hyde Park, N.Y.: University Books, 1967.

Saltman, Jules, *Marijuana and Your Child*. New York: Grosset and Dunlap, 1970.

Schachter, S., "Cognitions and Response to Marihuana," *Advances in Experimental Social Psychology*, 1:76–79, 1964.

Simmons, Jerry L., ed., *Marihuana, Myths and Realities*. New York: Brandon House, 1967.

Simon, W. E., *et al.*, "A Comparison of Marijuana Users and Nonusers on a Number of Personality Variables," *Journal of Consulting and Clinical Psychology*, 42(6):917–918, 1974.

Smith, David E., *The New Social Drug*. Englewood Cliffs, N.J.: Prentice-Hall, 1970.

Solomon, David, *The Marihuana Papers*. New York: Bobbs-Merrill, 1966.

Surface, William, *The Poisoned Ivy*. New York: Coward McCann, 1968.

Tauro, G. J., "Marihuana and Relevant Problems of 1969," *American Criminal Law Quarterly*, 7:174–194, 1969.

United States Department of Health, Education, and Welfare, *Marijuana and Health*. Washington, D.C.: U.S. Government Printing Office, 1971.

Way, Walter, *The Drug Scene*. Englewood Cliffs, N.J.: Prentice-Hall, 1970.

Zunin, L. M., "Marijuana: the Drug and the Problem," *Military Medicine*, 134:104–110, 1969.

MARIJUANA TERMINOLOGY

Bad trip	Unpleasant experience, usually caused by panic reaction after taking a drug
Bar	A solid block of marijuana with sugar or Coca-Cola to make it stick together
Bong	Smoking instrument designed for maximal inhalation and minimal smoke loss
Bummer	An anxiety-producing trip on marijuana, LSD, etc.; to some, a bummer is considered less intense than a "bad trip"
Burned	Got phony drugs
Busted	Arrested for taking drugs
Chippying	Using drugs irregularly
Connect	Find a source and buy drugs
Crash	Fall asleep after a prolonged high
Dabble	Use drugs irregularly
Dealer	Seller or pusher of drugs
Euphoria	An exaggerated sense of well-being
Glow	High, euphoria
Gold leaf	High-grade marijuana
Grass	Marijuana

Grasshopper	One who uses marijuana
Hash	Hashish, pure resin from the cannabis plant; most potent source of THC, next to its liquid concentrate, hash oil
Hay	Marijuana
Hemp	Marijuana
Jag	Under the influence of marijuana
Joint	Marijuana cigarette
Kilo	A kilogram (2.2 pounds) brick of marijuana
Lid	A street measure of marijuana, about an ounce; makes up into about 40 marijuana cigarettes, depending on how clean it is
Manicure	Marijuana of high grade; or (as a verb) to remove the stems and seeds from marijuana leaves
Maryjane	Marijuana
Matchbox	A street measure of marijuana, about 0.2 ounce; makes up into about 6–7 marijuana cigarettes
Mexican brown	Good grade of marijuana from Mexico
Nickel bag	$5 packet of marijuana, same quality as matchbox
On	Under the influence of marijuana
Pot	Marijuana
Quarter bag	1 ounce of marijuana, sold for $25
Rap	Communicate, speak with rapport
Reefer	Marijuana cigarette
Roach	Marijuana cigarette butt
Roach holder	Matchbook cover, toothpick, hairpin, or other device used to hold the last bit of a marijuana cigarette so it can be smoked
Rope	Marijuana
Score	Find and buy marijuana
Seed	Marijuana cigarette butt
Stash	Hidden supply of marijuana or other drug
Stoned	Under the influence of drugs
Sweet Lucy	Resinous part of marijuana dissolved in wine
Tall	Being high or stoned
Texas tea	Marijuana
THC	Tetrahydrocannabinol, the active ingredient in marijuana and hashish which causes psychogenic reactions
Toke	A puff or drag on a marijuana cigarette
Toke pipe	Small, short-stemmed marijuana pipe
Weed	Marijuana

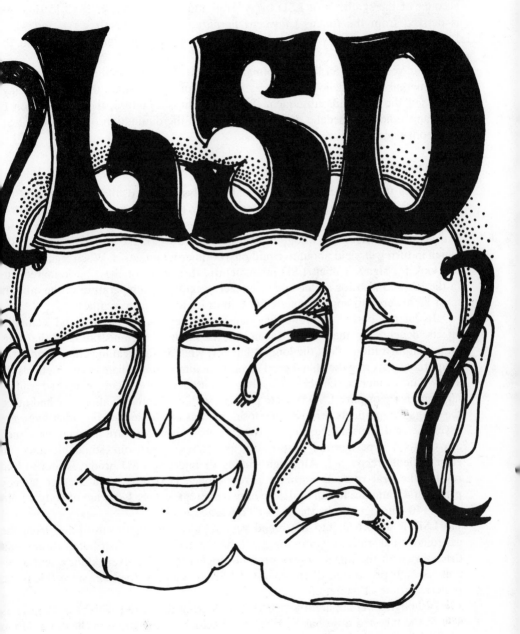

INTRODUCTION TO LSD

A century of research into the chemistry of ergot alkaloids preceded the first writte account of the synthesis of LSD by A. Stoll and A. Hofmann in 1943 [59]. Ergo is derived from the fungus *Claviceps purpurea,* which parasitizes rye and whea kernels, and from some varieties of morning glory plants containing lysergic acid, th precursor of LSD.

Four years after Stoll and Hofmann's report, Stoll reported the accidental an experimental psychedelic experiences of Hofmann [58]. Since that time we hav witnessed the ebb and subsequent flow of the hippie culture, the classification o LSD and other psychedelic drugs as illegal, and the diminution of interest in LSI as a front-page story.

Pharmacology

Ingredients used in the synthesis of LSD are lysergic acid, diethylamine, and tri fluoroacetic acid. Lysergic acid is controlled by the Federal Drug Administration but illicit manufacturers also produce it in clandestine labs using *Claviceps purpurec* and mannitol. About one kilogram of lysergic acid will make one-half kilo of LSD which in turn will yield about five million 100-microgram doses. When legal authori ties look for signs of illicit LSD manufacture, they look for these basic ingredient in the lab and also for an ice-cream freezer because the temperature of the mixtur must be lowered to approximately 20°F in order to complete synthesis.

Its latency period, the time that elapses between taking the drug and feeling it effects, depends on the amount taken and the mode of administration of the drug Oral administration offers the longest latency, while intrathecal injection (under th membranes covering the spinal cord) causes an almost immediate onset of effects. Ir 1974 San Francisco General Hospital admitted eight patients who had sniffec large amounts of pure LSD tartrate powder, within 15 minutes after they had taker the drug. Two patients arrived comatose, one was catatonic, and the other five were psychotic and hyperactive. Supportive care was given for various symptoms such as vomiting, hyperthermia, respiratory arrest, upper gastrointestinal bleeding; all eight patients recovered. Although sniffing or injecting LSD produces more rapid results, the oral route is normally taken. Cohen [13] reports an average latency period of 45 minutes for an oral dose of two micrograms per kilogram of body weight (i.e., 140 micrograms in the 70 kg "reference man").

LSD is absorbed into the blood very rapidly, and upon absorption from the gastrointestinal mucosa (oral administration), it is rapidly distributed throughout the body, with the highest concentrations appearing in the liver, kidney, and adre-nals. A high proportion of the ingested LSD is found in the bile, since this is the preferred route of excretion.

Although LSD apparently crosses the blood-brain barrier with ease, as little as 1% of the ingested dose has been found to actually concentrate in the brain. Upon examining levels of LSD concentration in various parts of the monkey brain,

Snyder and Reivich [54] found the highest concentrations in the pituitary gland and pineal gland, but high concentrations were also found in the hypothalamus, the limbic system, and the auditory and visual reflex areas. Surprisingly low concentrations were found in the cortex, cerebellum, and the brainstem. This information helps to explain the electrical storms found (via depth electrodes) to occur in areas within the limbic system in LSD subjects, while electroencephalogram records of other brain areas showed no change [43].

Physiological effects, tolerance, and dose

If LSD is ingested, a number of physiological effects will become increasingly apparent as the latency period comes to an end. Among these effects are a tingling in the hands and feet, a feeling of numbness, nausea (and sometimes vomiting), anorexia (lack of appetite), a flushed appearance, sensations of chilliness, and dilation of the pupils (mydriasis). Mydriasis, along with increased heart rate, body temperature, blood pressure, and blood sugar level, persists throughout the "psychic" period characterizing the LSD trip, but the other physiological effects subside. Hoffer and Osmond [27] state that the extent of pupil dilation is one of the most effective ways to determine LSD activity in subjects; thus mydriasis is one means of identifying an LSD tripper (the behavioral effects, however, may be more obvious).

Jarvik et al. [31–34] and other investigators have found that LSD impairs intellectual processes; the subject cannot or will not perform given tasks, has difficulty in concentrating, and shows an overall air of confusion. All types of psychological tests (perceptual, cognitive, and motor) given by Jarvik and his colleagues have revealed impairment by LSD.

Tolerance to LSD develops quite rapidly. Abramson et al. [2] have shown that there is a quite noticeable decrease in subjective symptoms when the same moderate dose is given daily for several days; hence, those who use LSD for "kicks" must either space their trips or take ever-increasing doses if they use it daily.

A standard dose of LSD for the average man is considered to be 100 micrograms, but dosages as high as 1500 micrograms have been reported in supervised medical treatment, and occasionally a chronic user will report taking dosages as high as 10,000 micrograms [13]. In addition to dosage, effects depend also on the frame of mind of the user and his or her personality and environment. To date, no deaths have been reported from overdoses of LSD in man.

Neurochemical action of LSD

LSD has various effects on the nervous system, but a delineation of exactly which chemical reactions cause the psychedelic reaction in man is still awaited.

It is known that LSD and a number of the other hallucinogens have in their basic chemical makeup a structure known as an *indole ring*. This indole ring is also part of the basic structure of serotonin, a neurohormone known to exist in brain structures, especially in the reticular area, the hypothalamus, and the limbic system.

Although research is contradictory and incomplete, this indole ring could play a part in the antagonistic action LSD has on serotonin, which may, in turn, play a part in the overall action of LSD in the brain.

LSD's *inhibition* of nerve impulses in various parts of the brainstem, visual system, and other brain areas makes it difficult to comprehend why typical alertness and arousal-type reactions occur in LSD subjects [7, 8, 25].

Hoffer and Osmond [27] have enumerated several ways (though these are not definitely substantiated by research) in which LSD may cause its characteristic effects: (a) by mimicking the amines such as norepinephrine, (b) by depleting amines from nerve endings, (c) by blocking the action of the amines, probably serotonin, and (d) by not allowing the release of histamine or serotonin.

THE ACID EXPERIENCE

In a supportive setting, the LSD user usually first shows signs of his trip by becoming extremely emotional. A minor remark or incident may set off an intense laughing or crying episode. Of all the senses, tactile sensitivity is most universally affected, and the most dramatic effects are those of hallucinations, although they are often absent.

As the drug begins to take hold, one of the first visual effects to occur is that of ever-changing colors and shapes of objects in the room, and the appearance of rainbowlike halos around lights. The senses are further affected, and synesthesia, a crossing of sense responses (hearing colors and seeing sounds), may occur. All this time may be spent in awe of the deepness of colors, the beauty of one object, the pureness of sound; but while LSD enhances visual and auditory perception, it also works on other central nervous system centers. Time and space perception are quite lost, and because of its stimulatory nature LSD permits many extra stimuli to enter thought processes. Sounds and sights may flash on and off, tripping thought processes that have been long forgotten.

If a large enough dose is taken, the tripper will begin to lose touch with the outside "concrete" world and begin to feel part of some greater living cosmos where ego boundaries have been erased. The ineffable nature of this feeling seems to parallel Maslow's "peak experience"—a feeling of "being one" with all things, an ecstasy of spirit. Especially in supportive settings, trippers report seeing divine figures, enchanting places, and other images of religiosity.

Thus, the trip itself gives insight into the great rise and fall of acid as the sacrament of the flower children of the 1960s.

LSD and spiritual search

The increase in use of the psychedelics (and marijuana) has roots deep into the American culture of the 1940s and 1950s. The country had emerged from a depression and entered a postwar boom. Parents strove to obtain the possessions they lacked in the depression days and vowed that their children would have the best of everything and be without worry of hunger and want. The "war babies" knew a greater security than many of their parents had known and experienced a new kind of freedom. Perhaps out of this very freedom and security grew the disregard for material wealth and the superficial life that many times accompanied it. Established practices were challenged in increasing numbers with increasing vigor, and a new movement was under way with an ethic of love, individual freedom, and personal honesty. McGlothlin [38] likened the young people of this movement to the early Christians: both groups preached a doctrine of love, rejection of earthly possessions, the game-free state that involved avoidance of pride and other aspects of vanity, and support from communal living. Even such superficial things as hair style and clothing were similar between the two groups. Also, like the early Christians, the individuals involved in this movement (who became known as hippies) were rejected by the established society.

During this time a Harvard professor by the name of Timothy Leary was discovering the religious wonders of psychedelic drugs and began making a case for their inclusion in religious ceremony. He wanted everyone to have religious experiences whereby they might learn the answers to four basic spiritual questions [35]:

1. The Ultimate-Power Question (What is the power that moves the universe?),
2. The Life Question (What is life?),
3. The Human-Destiny Question (What is man's role?), and
4. The Ego Question (What is my role?).

These questions were being asked by the youthful revolutionaries who were turning away from organized religion to a religion of their own. LSD and marijuana became the drugs of choice as both have been linked to a passive, introspective lifestyle.

In 1967 a group of San Francisco Bay Area physicians who were concerned with the effects of psychedelic drugs sponsored a conference on "The Religious Significance of Psychedelic Drugs" in which legal, social, and cultural aspects of the psychedelic religious movement were discussed [60]. At this meeting one of the panelists, Reverend Laird Sutton, focused on certain cultural and spiritual vacuums that he felt were instrumental in the hippie movement. The main cultural vacuum was that of the love ethic having been replaced by a duty ethic in the larger society, and he felt that it was this vacuum that the hippies were trying to fill. Sutton's religious vacuum was many-faceted, but highly insightful into the 1960s culture. He pointed out that in the United States at that time there were but a few acceptable forms of worship and that society felt a profound distrust of mysticism and a secrecy toward man's spirituality. He also stated that the education of most young people lacked certain periods of time that were set aside specifically for individual religious development, and that there were few opportunities in our society for one to engage in philosophical or religious search as to the meaning of life and existence. In addition, he pointed out a paucity of religious literature dealing with the psychedelic or spiritual experience. For many in the hippie movement these served as motivations for examining a new way of life and a more profound type of spiritual experience than was available in the name of Methodism, Catholicism, or Judaism.

At this conference an air of optimism was apparent—there was a general feeling that this new love ethic could spread and give our society new life.

Such optimism was not seen by Huston Smith, an MIT professor, who in 1966, even before the great hippie upsurge, predicted that the whole movement would not have a religious impact because it did not have an established, stable community or church; it had no guidelines for behavior; it failed to formulate an integrated social philosophy demonstrating how the psychedelic experience influenced ongoing life; and it failed to convince the established society that what it was experiencing was meaningful [53]. Smith did prophesy the demise of the large hippie communities such as the Haight-Ashbury community of 1967–1968, but we see vestiges of this original movement in communes throughout the world, and, in general, an age of greater awareness was stimulated by the movement.

The death of the Hippie-Haight lay at the hands of the very people involved there, for the Haight (and other specific communities such as Greenwich Village in New York) was a mixture of all people. Yablonski [66] described it as a mixture of "High Priests" (the philosophers of the scene), novitiates, or the army of aspirants, and finally the "plastic hippies" who were subdivided into groups of hippie drug addicts, teenyboppers, severely emotionally disturbed people, and a miscellany of "others." Yablonski, in his continental visit into the hippie community during its peak, saw the movement as composed of a few philosophers (10–15%), a larger group of true seekers (35%), and then a group of fringe people who were part-time dropouts, teenage runaways, or drug addicts who used the movement as a form of immunity from established society. Also from his experiences with and in the movement, Yablonski estimated that 20% of the total number involved were seriously emotionally disturbed young people who also were using the movement as a place to hide or a method of dealing with their psychoses.

This breakdown of the characters involved in the movement facilitates the understanding of why large communities died out. There were large numbers of individuals who were not committed to a deep philosophy and were rather like leeches drawing their lifeblood from the community. The underlying philosophy of the movement was to "do your own thing," and when antinomianism is the rule, we find (as Noyes, the founder of the Oneida colony, one of the longest-lived communes in the United States, did in the 1800s) that without rules a community is faced with three major disruptive forces: lethargy, antiorganization or anarchy, and sexual irresponsibility. These problems also appeared in the many communes that grew out of the counterculture movement of the 1960s and caused their early demise. Groups of individuals who sought to remove themselves from the rules of the "Establishment" failed in their efforts when they rejected organization.

And so the strong, concentrated movement of the 1960s has become a low-key, more personal search for human interaction based on honesty, love, and individual freedom, and the psychedelic drug scene has subsided in a similar manner.

No longer do the media romanticize the "trip" or its users; the psychedelic clichés have been replaced by new jargon; and the chromosome issue is taken over by marijuana and other more popular drugs. But the psychedelics are still being used, and on some college campuses there has been a constant, modest increase in their use during the 1970s [20].

Deceit and dangers

Surveys show that many street users think they are purchasing mescaline, peyote, psilocybin, or other organics that have become popular along with organic gardening and "health" food; but there is good reason to believe that they are actually buying acid, PCP, or some other more easily manufactured hallucinogen. There are many synthetics on the street market (STP, DMT, PCP, for example) that are being sold along with acid. Some are wild mixtures of these substances and/or other adulterants [9]. A study conducted by the University of Maryland School of Pharmacy [63] concerning street drug rip-offs showed that street acid generally was LSD: but out of 57 samples of proposed mescaline, 43 were LSD and only one was mescaline, while the other 13 samples included PCP, sucrose, and nicotine. Nearly all the other 45 samples proposed to be peyote, mescaline, psilocybin, or a mixture thereof proved to be LSD, also. Supporting evidence also comes from the Haight-Ashbury Free Clinic which found that 90% of all hallucinogen samples that they analyzed were substances other than what they were claimed to be [51]. This street drug deceit could be a hazard to those who expect one kind of drug reaction, but find themselves in an entirely different experience. Since the intensity and length of the trip depends on drug and dosage, the street buyer must exercise caution.

Although there has been an atmosphere of adventure surrounding the psychedelics, they are not without drawbacks. Two dangers involved in psychedelic use that were given a great deal of coverage in the early days of the hippie world were bad trips and flashbacks. These phenomena are related in that both probably involve the memory process and other intricacies of the central nervous system. Cohen [13] estimates that about 0.1% of normal individuals who take LSD under favorable laboratory conditions suffer serious reactions. Although the percentage is small, it would be negligent to omit the dangers that are inherent in the use of psychedelic drugs (with LSD as the prototype in our discussion).

The bad trip, or "freakout" as it once was called, could be triggered by various stimuli. The panic that might result from loss of time-space perception, the acute physiological reactions of heart palpitation, chilliness, and nausea, or mere confusion from the experience could initiate a bad trip. Trippers might get so involved in their pseudohallucinations (true hallucinations occur only with high dosages and/or a very supportive setting) that they can no longer extricate themselves from their environment. If they panic, lose self-control and judgment, and perhaps become incoherent or violent, they and those around them are in a potentially dangerous situation. Since LSD wears off gradually over a period of 10–16 hours, the user cannot come out immediately except with the use of an anti-LSD drug such as chlorpromazine. However, the use of such a drug should be weighed against the possible harmful effects of subsequent psychological problems and a higher probability of flashbacks. In many, if not most, cases, a person on a bad trip can be talked back into a calm state; violence and restraint should be used only as a last measure. One should never tell the tripper in this condition that he or she has lost his or her mind or damaged it permanently, because the tripper is already in a frightened, irrational state and unable to think calmly or to use logical reasoning.

The bad trip can occur from an unexpected upsurge of memories that are normally repressed. It is not wise for a person with an unstable personality to take LSD, because the problems he or she has during an undrugged state may be amplified by LSD. It is not known exactly how LSD works, but it appears that normal selective damping of incoming stimuli no longer takes place and electrical storms occur in various parts of the brain. Convulsive seizures have even been known to occur during an LSD trip [11, 61].

A danger to many initial users is an intense expectation that doors will open, truth will be seen, and the soul will truly be enlightened. Expectation may be so great that anything short of an extremely moving experience may induce depression and a bad trip may ensue.

Another acute psychological danger is that ego boundaries may disappear; for example, the floor may seem to become part of the tripper, and to step on the floor may evoke bodily pain within the tripper. Ego may be inflated to heights beyond compare—to pure omnipotence—or to extreme lows, where suicide may seem to be the only way out. (However, this occurrence is quite rare.)

Thinking loses its logic. There is a danger that users will begin to be fanatically set on illogical "truths" which come to them during an LSD trip. They may believe they can read minds, can transmit ESP messages, can will themselves to do anything, or can even make themselves believe beyond a doubt that others are trying to kill them or are fiendishly plotting against them. Because of this inability to separate idea from reality during the drugged state, a striking number of LSD users strongly believe in magic [51].

It appears that mental stability, a supportive environment, and a good frame of mind upon going into an LSD experience are necessities. Taking LSD in an angry or apprehensive mood has been shown to increase the likelihood of a bad trip [47]; hence, one should never be given LSD when he or she is unwilling to take the drug. Above all, LSD should never be given to individuals who are unaware that they are taking it, for they will not be prepared for the effects, which sometimes even chronic users cannot handle.

Flashbacks

A well-publicized chronic reaction to LSD is the flashback, and although this phenomenon does not occur with everyone who takes LSD, it is impossible to tell who will experience it. It seems to occur most often in cases where the user has had a

ıad trip [47]. Feelings of paranoia, unreality, and estrangement are often experi-
ınced in the flashback [18] along with distorted visual perceptions and anesthesias
ır paresthesias (prickly or tingling sensations) creeping over the body [47]. It has
ıeen shown that the body rids itself of LSD quite completely in about 48 hours, so
ıow the body can react in an LSD-induced manner after that time has lapsed is
ı question still to be answered. Fischer [19] attributes the flashback experience to
ı "stateboundness" which is initiated by a stimulus identical to one previously
ıxperienced. An example of this is the sudden reflection or reliving of an experi-
ınce with a parent upon smelling their perfume or pipe tobacco. Experienced drug
ısers can sometimes cause a flashback by setting the environment that surrounded
ıhem in a previous experience; this is called a "free trip," for it occurs without the
ıse of a drug. Those who do not use drugs experience the same "free trip" when
ıhey have a moving memory of a happy experience.

Flashbacks have been known to last from a few minutes to several hours, to
ıccur one in a month or several times a day, up to 18 months after LSD use [18],
and to happen in many different settings. It has been found that other drugs may
trigger a flashback, and flashbacks frequently occur while one is driving or going
to sleep [47]; thus it would seem that they occur during a time when the reticular
formation is not forwarding a large number of stimuli into the cortex. This may
permit random thoughts or an overriding influence of any one thought or stimulus
to trigger a statebound experience. Flashbacks can be set off by stressful situations,
but may occur at nonstressful times as well.

There appear to be three kinds of flashbacks: perceptual (seeing colors, hearing sounds of the original experience), somatic (experiencing tingling sensations,
heart palpitations, etc.), and emotional (reliving of depressive, anxious, or otherwise emotional thoughts that may have been triggered by the initial trip). The first
two usually elicit reactions of panic, fear, and hysteria in those who do not understand the nature of them, but the third type may be the most dangerous because
the persistent feelings of fear, remorse, loneliness, or other emotions that might
occur may lead to extreme depression or suicide.

Chronic psychosis

Another psychological danger is that of prolonged psychosis or neurosis resulting
from LSD use. This is not a flashback, but is a continuing problem after the LSD
experience. Paranoiac and schizophreniform psychoses have been seen to occur
as a result of LSD, and the conditions have continued after the intoxication has
worn off [23]. Severe depression accompanying these psychoses has been thought
to be the cause of homicidal and suicidal actions that have followed.

The chromosome issue

A review of current research reveals numerous studies that report LSD's potential
for causing chromosomal breaks. Although the significance of such breaks has not

been definitely established, they have been found to occur in barley seeds [48], in animal and human white blood cells [14, 17, 30], in cells of a fetus conceived by users of LSD [62], and in a fetus exposed to LSD after conception [3]. In the last case some fetuses were deformed, while others were not [3, 4, 28]. Researchers have found meiotic chromosome change in mice directly exposed to high doses of LSD, and have indicated that LSD may have serious effects on size of litters, congenital malformations, and frequency of leukemia and other neoplastic disease (that is, diseases involving growth of nonfunctional tissue) [49].

On the other hand, there are numerous studies that report no cytogenic effects (harmful effects on the cells) and no teratogenic effects (harmful effects on the fetus) in rodents and rabbits [15, 44, 65] and in man [24]. In studying white blood cells, Bender and Sankar [6] reported finding no such harmful effects in young schizophrenic children and, although the children were not studied until 20 to 48 months after exposure to LSD (during which time circulating lymphocytes may have been naturally replaced), the researchers attach particular significance to the fact that these children received up to 150 micrograms daily for two to three years. Similar results have also been reported by Loughman et al. [37] and Sparkes et al. [57].

Research in this area has come a long way in a comparatively short time, from the in vitro studies of Cohen et al. [10] in 1967 to the present in vivo studies. The complexity of the chromosome issue and the sophistication of the research tends to be somewhat confusing to the lay reader. Caution should be exercised in reading, analyzing, and comparing studies. Pitfalls such as method of analyzing breaks, method of subject selection (possibility of other drug contamination), type of experimental animal, weight of animal, purity of LSD used (pure chemical, dry LSD mixed with saline, street mixtures), time of examination after exposure to LSD, and probably most important, amount of LSD per kilogram body weight must be considered. Further consideration must be given to the type of teratogenic or cytogenic effect being studied. Chromosome breakage is of doubtful importance unless the germ cells are affected. Dishotsky et al. [15] point out, however, that many reports of chromosome damage have come from studies in which subjects have ingested illicit (not pure) LSD, and therefore, the harmful effects observed may have stemmed from adulteration substances rather than from the LSD. These same researchers also pointed out that at this time there is no evidence that LSD is a carcinogen or a mutagen.

Although researchers have no control over interpretations of their work by readers and news reporters, they should clearly caution their readers against extending their findings to situations not covered by physical and/or statistical controls. An illustration of this point was put forth by Hoey [26], who reported the response of ten lay friends to a nonconclusive case study of the cytogenic and teratogenic effects of LSD. Nine individuals interpreted the article as proving that LSD was responsible for the condition; one did not. We do not desire fewer research reports, and neither did Hoey, for research alone holds the answer to this question. However, caution should be exercised in reporting and interpreting these studies. The research papers on the potential dangers of LSD are too numerous and too

ell executed to disregard; however, at this time, condemnation of LSD use in
erms of physiological damage may be premature.

LSD use in psychotherapy

LSD has been used with limited success in psychotherapy. It must be understood
that, where found successful, the drug has been only a tool, just as a scalpel is a
tool. The scalpel, in the hands of a competent surgeon, can be used to benefit the
patient, but in the hands of others it can be a dangerous object. Therapeutic use of
LSD has not increased greatly over the years because of its limited success, legal
aspects, difficulty in procuring the drug, adverse reactions to the drug (even in a
controlled environment, bad trips can and do occur), and the problem of rapid
tolerance buildup in the patient.

LSD therapy has been tried by psychotherapists to help resolve various problems of their patients. It has had limited use in cases of alcoholism [41, 64], autism
[1, 5], paranoia and schizophrenia [21], and various other mental and emotional
disorders. Results of these uses have ranged from no improvement to complete
cure, but the largest percentage lies in the "slightly improved" category [16]. LSD
does not work for every therapist or every patient. When the drug does assist in the
improvement of a patient, it is a combination of patient, therapist, and drug, all
working together, that effects the cure.

When the beneficial effects of therapy are presented as a rationale for using the
drug in a nonmedical setting, one must realize that (a) the argument is based on
therapy with limited use and limited success, and (b) the question is one of *psychedelic therapy* as opposed to *psycholytic therapy*. Psycholytic therapy, the use of
LSD in a medical setting, calls for a low dosage (50–70 micrograms) administered
repeatedly over a long period of time. This low dosage appears to facilitate recall,
catharsis, abreaction, and other patient reactions that may aid in psychoanalysis.
As one can see, this is *not* the nontherapeutic LSD trip, where a larger dose is taken
and stronger reactions occur. Therefore, in rationalizing the nontherapeutic use of
LSD, one cannot cite the beneficial effects of psycholytic therapy, because this use
of LSD is quite different from street use in dosage and in effects.

Psychedelic therapy, which is used on occasion, is a specialized form of intensive therapy on a "one-shot" basis. A dose of 200 micrograms or more is used to
create a typical LSD experience, in which it is hoped that the patient will "find
himself" [42]. This type of therapy is used with patients who have a basic loss of
self-respect, self-esteem, and self-image, in the hope that the drug experience will
allow them to accept themselves once again. This experience must be preceded by
extensive therapeutic preparation for several weeks prior to the therapy session. The
setting must be extremely supportive—special music, lighting, pictures, etc., are
used—and, most important, a trained therapist must constantly be with the patient
during the 10- to 12-hour trip, shaping, directing, and guiding the trip. The therapist provides reassurance, averts anxiety, and is responsible for the success of the
experience. The session is followed up with supportive therapy to help redirect the
patient.

Not all sessions of psychedelic therapy produce effective results, and bad trip are known to occur in therapy as well as in street use [16, 21, 47].

Creativity

Because creativity stems from mood, perception, thought, and other workings of the mind, it is not easily judged; it is therefore difficult to determine whether LSD might enhance creativity.

LSD subjects have expressed the feeling of being more creative during the LSD experience, but the acts of drawing and painting during a trip are hindered by the motor effects of LSD and the products of creative effort under the influence of LSD largely prove to be inferior to those produced prior to the drug experience. Paint ings done in LSD-creativity studies have been reported as reminiscent of schizo phrenic art.

Harman et al. [22] found that a very light dose of mescaline (equivalent to 5 micrograms of LSD) proved helpful to a select group of engineers, scientists, and administrators who had specific problems that they could not solve before the drug experience. A majority of these subjects developed solutions to their problems after the drug experience. Whether or not they could have arrived at a similar solution in a "brainstorming" session or some other nondrug experience is impossible to say However, these were highly select, competent subjects who apparently possessed a certain degree of creativity before the drug experience.

McGlothlin et al. [39] tested 24 college students and found, through the use of creativity, attitude, and anxiety tests, that three LSD sessions (200-microgram doses) had no objective effect of enhanced creativity six months later. However many of the subjects said that they felt they were more creative. This paradox is noted in many areas of LSD study—subjects feel that they have more insights, are more creative, have more answers to life's questions, but do not demonstrate them objectively. Their overt behavior is not modified and these new insights are short lived unless they are reinforced by modified behavior.

In general, it has been found that LSD subjects report a greater interest in art and music after an LSD experience, and this greater awareness of the arts may give rise to some of the subjective feelings of creativity that have been reported.

The literature reveals that outstanding drug researchers, such as Hoffer and Osmond [27] and Cohen [12], feel that LSD does not enhance creativity in a non creative mind. The drug may alter electrical patterns so that sensations are different and thus evoke a new idea from existing knowledge. A person who does not know music will not become a pianist by taking LSD; he may become more interested in music, however.

OTHER HALLUCINOGENS

All hallucinogens produce similar reactions in the human body, but the intensity of the reaction varies among the different drugs. The preceding discussion of the

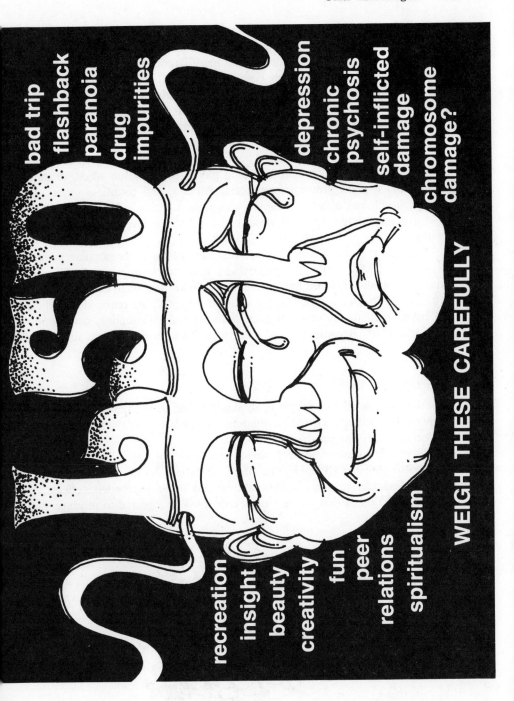

LSD

bad trip
flashback
paranoia
drug
impurities

depression
chronic
psychosis
self-inflicted
damage
chromosome
damage?

recreation
insight
beauty
creativity
fun
peer
relations
spiritualism

WEIGH THESE CAREFULLY

psychotherapeutic use of LSD gives an idea of the difference between the less i
tense reactions produced by a 50-microgram dose and the typical LSD trip caus
by a dose of 200 micrograms or more. The difference in intensity of the other h:
lucinogens parallels this type of continuum. It is found that an oral dose of C
milligram (100 micrograms) of LSD produces effects in humans comparable
the psychedelic effects produced by 10 milligrams of psilocybin or PCP, 200 mil
grams of DMT, or 400 to 800 milligrams of mescaline [12, 36, 50].

Hallucinogens that have seen high abuse, other than LSD, are mescalir
psilocybin, DMT, STP, and PCP. There are so many hallucinogens of minor pop
larity, such as nutmeg, certain morning glory seeds, jimson weed, ibogaine (o
tained from a plant grown in equatorial Africa), and countless others that tir
and space will not allow a complete description of each; however, the effects
these are very similar to those described for LSD, if large enough doses of the
are taken.

There is the ever-present danger for users of the more popular hallucinoge
(mescaline, DMT, STP, and psilocybin) that street supplies of these drugs a
quite often mislabeled and misrepresented, as was mentioned earlier in the chapte

LSD has been described in detail in this chapter; the remainder of the chapt
will be devoted to the other popular hallucinogens: mescaline, psilocybin, DM'
STP, and PCP. Because nitrous oxide can cause hallucinatory states, it is al
included.

Mescaline (and peyote)

Mescaline is one of the principal alkaloids found in the peyote cactus (Fig. 5.1
(*Lophophora williamsii*) and is apparently responsible for the visual hallucinatio
that occur when one eats peyote.

Peyote intoxication differs somewhat from mescaline intoxication becau:
peyote also contains alkaloids other than mescaline. A dose of 300–600 milligran
of mescaline can produce hallucinations and other psychedelic effects, wherea
more than 50 times that amount of peyote must be ingested to produce similar r

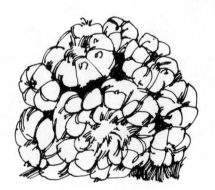

Fig. 5.1 The peyote cactus.

tions. Duration of effects for mescaline is 5 to 12 hours, but longer periods have en reported [36, 50].

Mescaline may be marketed as a powder, as a gelatin capsule, or in liquid rm, thus making it possible to sniff, ingest, or mainline the substance. However, is reported that most mescaline is taken orally. Peyote is taken orally in the form mescal buttons, the brown, dried crowns of the cactus. These buttons are either 1ewed or sucked to extract the hallucinogenic substances within.

Peyote is the only drug of its kind that is legal in the United States. This is 1e to the fact that it is part of the ritual ceremony performed by the Indians of the ative American Church of North America, a religious group of nearly a quarter illion members, which preaches brotherly love, high morality, and abstention om alcohol. However, the drug must be used strictly for religious ceremony, and eyotists must deal with legal suppliers for their drug.

The peyote ceremony usually consists of an all-night gathering inside the cere-1onial meeting place, where the worshippers sit in a circle around a fire. Peyote is 1ken and works its effects as the worshippers are led in prayer, chanting, and 1editation by a "road-man." The meeting ends in the morning with a communal 1eal [45, 46].

Peyote intoxication first brings on a feeling of contentment and hypersensitiv-y, then one of nervous calm during which visual hallucinations are apt to occur. rilliant flashes of color, defying description, are seen prior to the visual hallucina-ons. It appears that visual hallucinations occurring from peyote ingestion follow pattern. First, geometric figures appear, then familiar scenes and faces, followed y unfamiliar scenes and objects. It is this visual phenomenon that makes peyote evered by peyotists—this is their way of communicating with their spirits.

If this drug (peyote) and its derivative (mescaline) were used only as re-gious objects, they would be of little concern. However, the use of these hallucino-ens has entered the pleasure-seeking world, and if they are taken in sufficient osage, their use and the problems they cause become similar to those described or LSD. Like LSD, no physical dependence on these drugs has been observed, but he need for further psychological gratification may provide the impetus for re-eated use. Tolerance to mescaline develops, as does cross-tolerance between 1escaline, LSD, and psilocybin.

silocybin

n 1958 A. Hofmann (who discovered the hallucinogenic effects of LSD) isolated silocybin, the hallucinogenic agent in *Psilocybe mexicana,* a small mushroom that rows in marshy places (Fig. 5.2). This mushroom has been used for centuries in eligious ceremonies. The Aztecs used it as a sacrament and to produce visions and allucinations.

This drug (along with another *Psilocybe mexicana* derivative, psilocin) also as fallen into street use as a psychedelic. It is available in powder or liquid form, nd a dose of 4–8 milligrams will produce effects similar to those of mescaline,

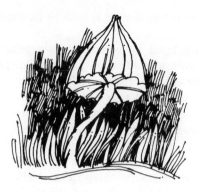

Fig. 5.2   The mushroom *Psilocybe mexicana,* from which psilocybin is produced.

including initial nausea, coldness of the extremities, and mydriasis, followed b
abrupt mood changes and visual hallucinations. The intoxication, lasting abou
eight hours, is followed by mental and physical depression, lassitude, and distor
tion of one's sense of time and space.

Psilocybin use has been shown to cause development of tolerance. No physi
cal dependence has been observed, but psychological dependence is a danger.

DMT

This hallucinogen has been labeled "the businessman's trip" because a 70-milli
gram dose will cause an onset of hallucinatory effects within two to five minutes
with the condition subsiding within half an hour to an hour.

This drug was originally obtained from seeds of *Piptadenia peregrina* an
Piptadenia macrocarpa, legumes that are found in the Caribbean Islands and i
South America. The natives of these areas pulverized the seeds and then inhalec
the substance as snuff through a tube.

DMT sold on the street now is a semisynthetic that is easily produced from
common materials (thus it is inexpensive and its street use is growing). It is very
similar in chemical structure to psilocin, the substance into which psilocybin i
converted in the body and which subsequently causes the psychedelic experience to
occur. It is usually smoked in a mixture of parsley, marijuana, tobacco, or tea

DMT (and its close chemical variant DET, diethyltryptamine) has not beer
found to cause physical dependence, but tolerance does develop, as may an intense
desire to continually repeat the experience.

STP

Psychotomimetic amphetamines are a group of amphetamines that produce hallucinogenic reactions along with the typical amphetamine reactions to be discussec
in Chapter 6. This group of psychoactive drugs is exemplified by DOM (di-
methoxymethylamphetamine), more popularly known as STP. The nickname STI

ems to have been derived from the popular motor oil additive "scientifically
eated petroleum" or from the words "serenity, tranquility, and peace."

As has been mentioned, STP is capable of producing typical LSD-type reac-
ons or amphetamine action, or both. As with most other drugs, the reaction de-
ends on the dose. In clinical studies reactions have been observed with doses vary-
ng from 2 to 14 milligrams, while street doses appear to be around 10 milligrams.
n a dosage continuum with other hallucinogenic compounds, STP is considered
o be about 100 times more potent than mescaline and about one-thirtieth as potent
s LSD [55].

Ingested doses of less than three milligrams produce heart rate increases, pu-
illary dilation, increase in systolic blood pressure, and increases in oral tempera-
ure. The experience at this dosage has been described as a mild euphoria. The
uration of reaction at low doses is from 8 to 12 hours, with peak reactions occur-
ing between the third and fifth hours [55].

With higher doses reactions may last from 16 to 24 hours. This duration may
e responsible for the high incidence of acute panic reactions associated with this
rug. In the extreme hyperactive condition, the even larger increases in heart rate,
lood pressure, and body temperature, along with pupillary dilation, an extremely
ry mouth, nausea, and profuse sweating, all seem to be endless. These effects are
ccompanied by LSD-type alterations in perception (such as enhancement of de-
ails), visual and auditory hallucinations (including blurred multiple images, dis-
orted shapes, and vibration of objects), and a slowed passage of time. The mind
ecomes flooded with a variety of irrelevant and incoherent thoughts, then becomes
bsolutely blank, exacerbating the feeling that one is going crazy [52, 56]. Also,
s is the case with LSD, flashbacks or recurrent reactions have been reported to
ccur, but no mechanism for this phenomenon has been substantiated [52].

The significance of these hallucinogenic breaks with reality is that they allow
or gross misinterpretation of the amphetaminelike somatic effects over an ex-
ended period of time. This combination of hallucinogenic and amphetaminelike
ffects appears to be the primary danger of psychotomimetic amphetamine com-
ounds like STP. The pharmacological effects have not been widely investigated,
ut the limbic system, the thalamus, and the hypothalamus seem to be affected.
These are the hypothesized sites of action because they are the sites of the greatest
ccumulation of STP in the brains of experimental animals [29].

PCP

The veterinary anesthetic phencyclidine (brand name, Sernyl) was used in the
arly 1960s as an anesthetic in humans, also; but upon emergence from Sernyl
nesthesia, many patients showed signs of disorientation, agitation, and/or psy-
hosis. These drawbacks necessitated its removal from human pharmacopoeia.
However, when psychogenic effects accompany a drug, there are those who are
willing to experiment with them. This and the apparent ease in manufacturing PCP
were responsible for the surge in its use across the country at a time when use of
ome of the other minor psychedelics had subsided.

PCP saw an upswing in 1967 on the west coast and in New York, and us
gradually covered the country; this has been a pattern seen with virtually all drug:
It came in tablet form as the Peace Pill, sprayed on parsley and called "Ang
Dust," mixed with marijuana as "Killer Weed," and in various other forms, th
majority of which were ingested or smoked. Reaction from intravenous injectio
was reported by the street world to be worse than a bad LSD trip and of a longe
duration.

Low dosages (7 mg orally) of PCP have effects that are similar to those of bai
biturate intoxication, whereas larger doses (12–15 mg) produce the psychedeli
reactions generally seen with high doses of LSD. At the high dose end of the scal
(15 mg and up) hallucinations and paranoid psychosis occur, and there are repori
of self-destructive behavior during intoxication at these dosages [40, 62].

Diazepam can be used to counteract severe psychoneurotic reactions or whe
there is risk of convulsions. Death from PCP overdose occurs due to convulsion
and/or depression of the respiratory centers.

Nitrous oxide

As a dental patient, one may have experienced the sudden onset of diminishe
ability to perceive pain while perhaps becoming statebound in a "double martin
high." Dentists who utilize nitrous oxide use a mixture that includes 40% oxygen
but when this drug is used by those seeking greater pleasure than the escape fron
a grating dentist drill, it may be inhaled as a pure gas. The major danger accom
panying the use of this drug is related to the concentration in which it is taken
If pure nitrous oxide is inhaled over a period of two to three minutes, anoxia wil
occur, which could give rise to serious physical effects such as organic brain dam
age, heart failure, or death from lack of oxygen.

Signs of anoxia can be observed by others—the nitrous oxide inhaler will be
come cyanotic ("turn blue"), muscles will twitch, and respiration rate and deptl
will increase. A rise in blood pressure also accompanies these outward signs. I
respiration becomes shallow or stops, the individual should be given resuscitative
measures immediately.

In general, low-dose, low-frequency nitrous oxide use, accompanied by oxyger
inhalation, is probably harmless, but because of the psychic effects, there is alway:
the possibility of psychological dependence in susceptible individuals.

REFERENCES

1. Abramson, H. A., ed., *The Use of LSD in Psychotherapy and Alcoholism.* India
napolis: Bobbs-Merrill, 1967.
2. Abramson, H. A., et al., "LSD: XVII. Tolerance and its Relationship to a Theory
of Psychosis," *Journal of Psychology,* 41:81, 1956.
3. Alexander, G. I., and B. E. Miles, "LSD: Injection Early in Pregnancy Produces Ab
normalities in Offspring of Rats," *Science,* 157:459–460, 1967.

4. Auerbach, R., and J. Rugowski, "LSD: Effect on Embryos," *Science,* 157:325–326, 1967.

5. Bender, L., *et al.,* "LSD and UML Treatment of Hospitalized Disturbed Children," *Recent Advances in Biological Psychiatry,* 5:84, 1963.

6. Bender, L., and D. V. S. Sankar, "Chromosome Damage Not Found in Leukocytes of Children Treated with LSD-25," *Science,* 159:749, 1968.

7. Boakes, R. J., *et al.,* "Antagonism of 5-Hydroxytryptamine by LSD 25 in the Central Nervous System: a Possible Neuronal Basis for the Actions of LSD 25," *British Journal of Pharmacology,* 40:202–218, 1970.

8. Bradley, P. B., and J. Elkes, "The Effects of Some Drugs on the Electrical Activity of the Brain," *Brain,* 80:77, 1957.

9. Cheek, P. E., and S. Newell, "Deceptions in the Illicit Drug Market," *Science,* 167:1276, 1970.

10. Cohen, M. M., *et al.,* "Chromosomal Damage in Human Leukocytes Induced by LSD," *Science,* 155:1417–1419, 1967.

11. Cohen, S., "A Classification of LSD Complications," *Psychosomatics,* 7:182–186, 1966.

12. Cohen, S., *The Drug Dilemma.* New York: McGraw-Hill, 1969.

13. Cohen, S., "A Quarter Century of Research with LSD," in J. T. Ungerleider, ed., *The Problems and Prospects of LSD.* Springfield, Ill.: Charles C. Thomas, 1968.

14. Dipaolo, J. A., H. M. Givelber, and H. Erwin, "Evaluation of Teratogenicity of LSD," *Nature,* 220:490–491, 1968.

15. Dishotsky, N., *et al.,* "LSD and Genetic Damage," *Science,* 172:431–440, 1971.

16. Ditman, K. S., and T. Moss, "The Value of LSD in Psychotherapy," in J. T. Ungerleider, ed., *The Problems and Prospects of LSD.* Springfield, Ill.: Charles C. Thomas, 1968.

17. Egozcue, J., S. Irwin, and C. A. Maruffo, "Chromosomal Damage in LSD Users," *Journal of the American Medical Association,* 204:122–126, 1968.

18. Fisher, D. D., "The Chronic Side Effects from LSD," in J. T. Ungerleider, ed., *The Problems and Prospects of LSD.* Springfield, Ill.: Charles C. Thomas, 1968.

19. Fischer, R., "The 'Flashback': Arousal-Statebound Recall of Experience," *Journal of Psychedelic Drugs,* 3(2):31–39, 1971.

20. Girdano, D. A., and D. D. Girdano, "Drug Usage Trends Among College Students," *College Student Journal,* 8:94–96, 1974.

21. Grof, S., "Use of LSD 25 in Personality Diagnostics and Therapy of Psychogenic Disorders," in H. A. Abramson, ed., *The Use of LSD in Psychotherapy and Alcoholism.* Indianapolis: Bobbs-Merrill, 1967.

22. Harman, W. W., *et al.,* "Psychedelic Agents in Creative Problem Solving: a Pilot Study," *Psychological Review,* 19:211, 1966.

23. Hatrick, J. A., and K. Dewhurst, "Delayed Psychosis Due to LSD," *Lancet,* 2:742–744, 1970.

24. Hecht, F., *et al.,* "LSD and Cannabis as Possible Teratogens in Man," *Lancet,* 2:1087, 1968.

25. Himwich, H. E., in L. Cholden, ed., *Proceedings of the Round Table on LSD and Mescaline in Experimental Psychiatry*. London: Grune and Stratton, 1956.

26. Hoey, J., "LSD and Chromosome Damage," *Journal of the American Medical Association*, 212:1707, 1970.

27. Hoffer, A., and H. Osmond, *The Hallucinogens*. New York: Academic Press, 1967

28. Hsu, L., L. Strass, and K. Herschorn, "Chromosome Abnormality in Offspring of LSD Users," *Journal of the American Medical Association*, 211:987–990, 1970.

29. Idanpaan-Heikkila, J. E., *et al.*, "Relation of Pharmacological and Behavioral Effects of a Hallucinogenic Amphetamine to Distribution in Cat Brain," *Science*, 196:1085–1086, 1969.

30. Irwin, S., and J. Egozcue, "Chromosomal Abnormalities in Leukocytes of LSD-25 Users," *Science*, 157:313–314, 1967.

31. Jarvik, M. E., "The Behavioral Effects of Psychotogens," in R. C. DeBold and R. C. Leaf, eds., *LSD, Man and Society*. Middletown, Conn.: Wesleyan University Press, 1967.

32. Jarvik, M. E., *et al.*, "Lysergic Acid Diethylamide (LSD-25): IV. Effect on Attention and Concentration," *Journal of Psychology*, 39:373, 1955.

33. Jarvik, M. E., *et al.*, "Lysergic Acid Diethylamide (LSD-25): VI. Effect on Recall and Recognition of Various Stimuli," *Journal of Psychology*, 29:443, 1955.

34. Jarvik, M. E., *et al.*, "Lysergic Acid Diethylamide (LSD-25): VIII. Effect on Arithmetic Test Performance," *Journal of Psychology*, 39:465, 1965.

35. Leary, T., "The Religious Experience: Its Production and Interpretation," *Journal of Psychedelic Drugs*, 3:76–86, 1970.

36. Lerner, M., and M. D. Katsiaficas, "Analytical Separations of Mixtures of Hallucinogenic Drugs," *Bulletin on Narcotics*, 21:47–51, 1969.

37. Loughman, W. D., *et al.*, "Leukocytes of Humans Exposed to LSD," *Science*, 158: 508–510, 1967.

38. McGlothlin, W. H., "Hippies and Early Christianity," *Journal of Psychedelic Drugs*, 1:24–37, 1968.

39. McGlothlin, W., *et al.*, "Long Lasting Effects of LSD on Normals," *Journal of Psychedelic Drugs* (Haight-Ashbury Medical Clinic, San Francisco), 3(1), 1970.

40. Munch, J. C., "Phencyclidine: Pharmacology and Toxicology," *Bulletin on Narcotics*, 26(4):17–19, 1974.

41. O'Reilley, P., and G. Reich, "Lysergic Acid and the Alcoholic," *Diseases of the Nervous System*, 23:331–334, 1962.

42. Osmond, H., "A Review of the Clinical Effects of Psychotomimetic Agents," *Annals of the New York Academy of Sciences*, 66:418, 1957.

43. Purpura, D. P., "Neurophysiological Actions of LSD," in R. C. DeBold and R. C. Leaf, eds., *LSD, Man and Society*. Middletown, Conn.: Wesleyan University Press, 1967.

44. Roux, C., *et al.*, "LSD: No Teratogenic Action in Rats, Mice and Hamsters," *Science*, 169:588–589, 1970.

45. Schultes, R. E., "The Plant Kingdom and Hallucinogens (Part I)," *Bulletin on Narcotics*, 21:3–16, 1969.

46. Schultes, R. E., "The Plant Kingdom and Hallucinogens (Part III)," *Bulletin on Narcotics*, 22:25–53, 1970.

47. Shick, J. F. E., and D. E. Smith, "Analysis of the LSD Flashback," *Journal of Psychedelic Drugs* (Haight-Ashbury Medical Clinic, San Francisco), 3(1), 1970.

48. Singh, M. P., *et al.*, "Chromosomal Aberrations Induced in Barley by LSD," *Science*, 169:491–492, 1970.

49. Skakkeblk, N. E., and J. Philip, "LSD in Mice Abnormalities in Meiotic Chromosomes," *Science*, 160:1248–1249, 1968.

50. Smith, D. E., ed., *Drug Abuse Papers*. Berkeley: University of California Press, 1969.

51. Smith, D. E., *Journal of Psychedelic Drugs*, Vol. 3, No. 1. San Francisco: Haight-Ashbury Free Medical Clinic, 1970.

52. Smith, D. E., "The Psychotomimetic Amphetamines with Special Reference to STP (DOM) Toxicity," *Journal of Psychedelic Drugs*, 2:73–85, 1970.

53. Smith, H., "Psychedelic Theophanies and the Religious Life," *Journal of Psychedelic Drugs*, 3(1):87–91, 1970.

54. Snyder, S. H., and M. Reivich, "Regional Location of Lysergic Acid Diethylamide in Monkey Brain," *Nature*, 209:1093, 1966.

55. Snyder, S. H., *et al.*, "DOM (STP): a New Hallucinogenic Drug," *American Journal of Psychiatry*, 125:113–120, 1968.

56. Snyder, S. H., *et al.*, "2,5-Dimethoxy-4-Methyl-Amphetamine (STP)—a New Hallucinogenic Drug," *Science*, 158:669–670, 1967.

57. Sparkes, R. S., J. Melnijk, and P. Bozzetti, "Chromosomal Effect *in vivo* of Exposure to LSD," *Science*, 160:1343–1345, 1968.

58. Stoll, A., "Lysergsaure-diathy-amid, ein Phantasticum aus der Mutterkorngruppe," *Schweizer Archiv für Neurologie und Psychiatrie*, 60:279, 1947.

59. Stoll, A., and A. Hofmann, "Partialsynthese von Alkaloiden von Typus des Ergobasins," *Helvetica chimica acta*, 26:944, 1943.

60. Symposium, "Psychedelic Drugs and Religion," *Journal of Psychedelic Drugs*, 1:45–71, 1968.

61. Ungerleider, J. T., "The Acute Side Effects from LSD," in J. T. Ungerleider, ed., *The Problems and Prospects of LSD*. Springfield, Ill.: Charles C. Thomas, 1968.

62. University of Maryland School of Pharmacy, "Phencyclidine: A Hazardous Drug of Abuse," unpublished, 1972.

63. University of Maryland School of Pharmacy, "Street Drug Rip Off," unpublished, 1973.

64. Van Dusen, W., *et al.*, "Treatment of Alcoholism with Lysergide," *Quarterly Journal of Studies on Alcohol*, 28:295–304, 1967.

65. Warkany, J., and E. Takacs, "LSD: No Teratogenicity in Rats," *Science*, 159:731–732, 1968.

66. Yablonski, L., *The Hippie Trip*. Baltimore: Penguin Books, 1973.

67. Zellweger, H., J. S. McDonald, and G. Abbo, "Is Lysergic-Acid Diethylamide a Teratogen?" *Lancet*, 2:1066–1069, 1967.

SUGGESTED READING

Abramson, H. A., ed., *The Use of LSD in Psychotherapy and Alcoholism.* Indianapolis Bobbs-Merrill, 1967.

Alexander, M., *The Sexual Paradise of LSD.* North Hollywood, Calif.: Brandon House 1967.

Alpert, R., and S. Cohen, *LSD.* New York: New American Library, 1967.

Bishop, M. G., *The Discovery of Love: a Psychedelic Experience with LSD–25.* New York: Dodd, Mead, 1963.

Blum, Richard H., *et al., The Utopiates: the Use and Users of LSD–25.* New York: Atherton, 1964.

Bowers, M., A. Chipman, A. Schwartz, and O. T. Dann, "Dynamics of Psychedelic Drug Abuse," *Archives of General Psychiatry,* 16:560–566, 1967.

Braden, William, *The Private Sea: LSD and the Search for God.* Chicago: Quadrangle Books, 1967.

Caldwell, William V., *LSD Psychotherapy.* New York: Grove Press, 1968.

Campbell, R. S., *et al.,* "The Hippie Turns Junkie: the Emergence of a Type," *International Journal of the Addictions,* 9(5):719–730, 1974.

Carter, Charles H., *et al.,* "Lysergic Acid Diethylamide and Chromosome Damage: its Controversy," *Journal of the Florida Medical Association,* 59:29–31, 1972.

Cashman, J., *The LSD Story.* Greenwich, Conn.: Fawcett Publications, 1966.

Cohen, S., *The Beyond Within: the LSD Story.* New York: Atheneum, 1967.

Dunlap, Jane, *Exploring Inner Space: Personal Experiences under LSD–25.* New York: Harcourt, Brace, and World, 1961.

Garfield, J. M., *et al.,* "Effects of Nitrous Oxide on Decision-Strategy and Sustained Attention," *Psychopharmacologia,* 42(1):5–10, 1975.

Hollister, L. E., *Chemical Psychosis: LSD and Related Drugs.* Springfield, Ill.: Charles C. Thomas, 1967.

Hyde, M. O., *Mind Drugs.* New York: McGraw-Hill, 1968.

Jaffe, Dennis T., "The Repression and Support of Psychedelic Experience," *American Journal of Orthopsychiatry,* 42:290, 1972.

Jacobs, K. W., "Asthmador: A Legal Hallucinogen," *International Journal of the Addictions,* 9(4):503–512, 1974.

Kalent, L., *Mushrooms, Molds, and Miracles.* New York: John Day, 1965.

Kluver, H., *Mescal and Mechanics of Hallucination.* Chicago: University of Chicago Press, 1966.

Leary, T. F., *The Psychedelic Experience: a Manual Based on the Tibetan Book of the Dead.* New Hyde Park, N.Y.: University Books, 1964.

Masters, R. E., and J. Houston, *Varieties of Psychedelic Experience.* New York: Holt, Rinehart, and Winston, 1966.

Matefy, R. E., *et al.,* "An Initial Investigation of the Psychedelic Drug Flashback Phenomenon," *Journal of Consulting and Clinical Psychology,* 42(6):854–860, 1974.

Pollard, J. C., L. Uhr, and E. Stern, *Drugs and Phantasy: the Effects of LSD, Psilocybin and Sernyl on College Students.* Boston: Little, Brown, 1965.

Roseman, Bernard, *LSD: the Age of Mind.* Hollywood, Calif.: Wilshire, 1966.

Roseman, Bernard, *The Peyote Story.* Hollywood, Calif.: Wilshire, 1966.

Sackler, A. M., *et al.,* "Acute Effects of Mescaline HCl on Behavior, Resistance, and Endocrine Function of Male Mice," *Experimental Medicine and Surgery,* 29:118–127, 1971.

Smart, R. E., *LSD in the Treatment of Alcoholism.* Toronto: University of Toronto Press, 1968.

Soloman, D., ed., *LSD, the Consciousness Expanding Drug.* New York: Putnam's, 1964.

Ungerleider, J. T., ed., *Problems and Prospects of LSD.* Springfield, Ill.: Charles C. Thomas, 1968.

Usdin, E., and D. H. Efron, *Psychotropic Drugs and Related Compounds.* Washington, D.C.: Department of Health, Education, and Welfare, 1967.

Weil, G. M., ed., *The Psychedelic Reader.* New York: University Books, 1965.

Wesson, R. G., *The Hallucinogenic Fungi of Mexico: an Inquiry into the Origins of the Religious Idea among Primitive Peoples.* Cambridge, Mass.: Botanical Museum of Harvard University, 1961.

Wolstenholme, G. E. W., and J. Knight, eds., *Hashish: its Chemistry and Pharmacology.* Boston: Little, Brown, 1965.

HALLUCINOGEN TERMINOLOGY

Acid	LSD (lysergic acid diethylamide)
Acidhead	Chronic user of LSD
Amine	A substance having an NH_2 group in its chemical structure
Bad trip	Unpleasant experience, usually from panic reaction, after taking a drug
Big chief	Mescaline
Big D	LSD
Buttons	Usable part of peyote cactus
Coming down	The period when the effects of a drug, especially LSD, begin to wear off
Cube	A cube of sugar containing LSD
DMT	Dimethyltryptamine; similar in structure to psilocybin, but altered synthetically
DOM	Dimethoxymethylamphetamine (STP)
Drop	Swallow
Experience	LSD-type trip
Factory	Place for the manufacture of illicit drugs

Freakout	Bad experience, or temporary psychotic reaction
Mescal	Peyote
Mike	Microgram (usually of LSD); equals one-millionth of a gram
PCP	Phencyclidine; a veterinary anesthetic with psychedelic potential
Score	Find and buy drugs
Setting	Proper environment to take drugs, especially hallucinogens
Sitter	A person who is experienced in the use of LSD and aids someone else through the experience
STP	Dimethoxymethylamphetamine (DOM), a synthetic hallucinogen; STP may stand for the motor oil additive "scientifically treated petroleum," or "serenity, tranquility, and peace."
Trip or tripping out	An experience with LSD or other hallucinogens

6 AMPHETAMINES AND OTHER STIMULANTS

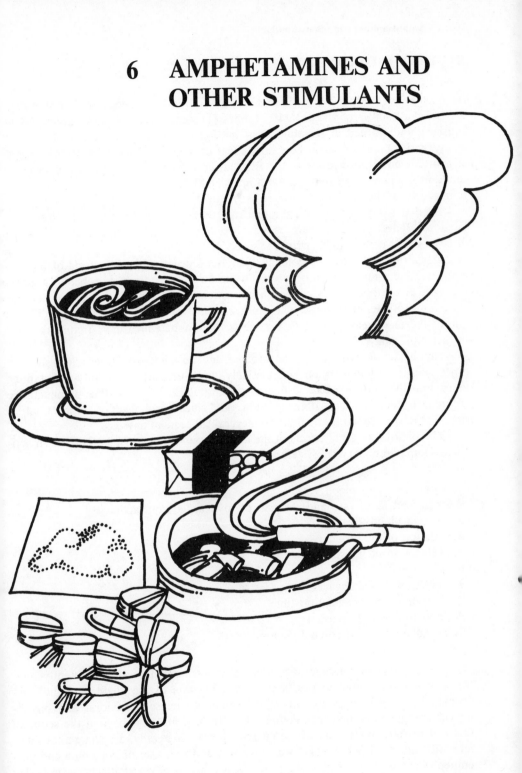

GENERAL INFORMATION

Amphetamines (Alpha-MethylPHenEThylAMINE) have been used as stimulant drugs for a number of years. In 1927 Alles [1] synthesized an amphetamine (Benzedrine) and learned of its stimulatory nature, which mimicked the action of the sympathetic nervous system. One of the first uses of Benzedrine was as a vasoconstrictor for nasal passageways—the Benzedrine Inhaler was introduced in 1932 by the Smith, Kline, and French Laboratories of Philadelphia. Later, this inhaler was removed from the market because of its frequent abuse.

Further study brought out the fact that there was an amphetamine closely related to Benzedrine; this was called Dexedrine. Further study also led to the discovery of methylamphetamine ("speed").

Dexedrine is of greater potency than Benzedrine, with the effects of methylamphetamine somewhere in between. Of the three, Dexedrine is probably of greatest medical use because even though its stimulatory effects on the central nervous system are greater than those of the other two, it offers fewer side effects. This is one of the main reasons that Dexedrine is the amphetamine most frequently used in diet pills today.

Amphetamines are quickly absorbed from the alimentary tract and also from other sites of administration. A relatively large proportion of an amphetamine taken into the body is excreted unchanged through the kidney; thus amphetamine is found in the urine soon after ingestion. And since metabolism of amphetamine is slow, the drug is found in the urine for several subsequent days.

The pharmacological effects of the amphetamines are typically those of an activated sympathetic nervous system:

1. Constriction of blood vessels
2. Increased heart rate and strength of myocardial contraction
3. Rise in blood pressure
4. Dilation of the bronchi
5. Relaxation of intestinal muscle
6. Mydriasis
7. Increased blood sugar
8. Shorter blood coagulation time
9. Increased muscle tension
10. Stimulation of the adrenal glands

These reactions combine to produce alertness, wakefulness, and attentiveness, all of which are characteristics of the *stress reaction* or the "fight or flight" syndrome. The mechanisms by which amphetamines cause behavioral and physiological changes have not been completely identified and it is beyond the scope of this text to fully analyze all of the current theory. Generally, amphetamines interfere with the synthesis, breakdown, turnover, and reuptake of dopamine and norepinephrine. Analysis of both the physiological and behavioral effects suggests that

amphetamine

IDENTIFICATION

Name	Nickname	Color and form		Normal dosage and use
Benzedrine (SKF*)	Bennies, peachies, truckdrivers, beans	Peach Maroon top, clear bottom with pink and white pellets	5 mg tab *Capsule*	5–30 mg daily for overweight or depression
Dexedrine (SKF*)	Dexies, Dex, brownies, hearts, oranges	Orange Brown top, clear bottom with orange and white pellets	5 mg tab *Capsule*	Up to 30 mg daily for obesity, depressive states, or alcoholism
Dexamyl (SKF*) 10 mg Dexedrine + 65 mg amobarbital OR 15 mg Dexedrine + 97 mg amobarbital "May be habit-forming"	Christmas trees	Green Green top, clear bottom with green and white pellets	5 mg tab *Capsule*	One capsule daily for diet control or depression
Methamphetamine hydrochloride	Meth, speed, crystal	*Desoxyn* (Abbot) white (5 mg) orange (10 mg) yellow (15 mg)		5–15 mg daily for depression 2.5 mg three times daily for obesity

* Smith, Kline, and French Laboratories

the site of amphetamine action is in the brainstem, closely related to the reticula
activating system (accounting for the effect of alertness) and in the hypothalamu
(accounting for behavioral reactions such as the elevation of mood).

Subjective effects of amphetamines include a feeling of euphoria, a sense o
well-being, a reduced hunger for food (anorexia), loquaciousness, hyperactivity
and a feeling of increased mental and physical power. A single dose (5–15 milli
grams) of amphetamine can produce these symptoms, and it has been found usefu
to administer the drug in emergencies when a person must keep awake and aler
over a longer than usual period of time (for instance, in the case of the astronauts
upon reentry into the earth's atmosphere). If wakefulness is prolonged more thar
1½ to 2 days, there is a high possibility that irritability, anxiety, and other un
toward effects will develop.

Therapeutic or medical use of the amphetamines is becoming very limited, anc
many people feel that there is little, if any, need for the further manufacture o
these drugs. A decrease in physician prescription and adverse reports from the
office of the Surgeon General led to the placement of amphetamines under schedule II of the Controlled Substances Act (i.e., drugs showing a high potential fo
abuse and limited medical use). In 1972 the Bureau of Narcotics and Dangerous
Drugs set quotas for the production of amphetamines at 22% of the 1971 figure
In 1973 additional quotas imposed on amphetamine production reduced production to about 11% of that produced in 1971, reported to be 10.2 tons of amphetamines and 5.4 tons of methamphetamine in that year.

THE USE OF AMPHETAMINES

Even though the effectiveness of amphetamines in the practice of medicine has
been questioned, prescriptions are still being written, mainly for the following purposes:

1. To treat minor depression. The depression treated with amphetamines should
   be a minor, short-lived one, since amphetamines are short-lasting, and a
   deeper depression may follow the waning of the drug's effects. Also, tolerance
   may build up with continuous use.

2. To control *symptoms* of narcolepsy. The stimulant nature of amphetamines
   counteracts the desire to sleep, but in no way helps to cure the condition.

3. To counteract the depressant action of barbiturates, alcohol, etc.

4. To suppress appetite (short-term use only, not effective in long-term weight
   reduction programs).

5. To control behavioral problems in children (hyperkinetic behavior).

6. To counteract or prevent sleep in persons required to perform or stay awake
   for long periods of time.

Misuse of amphetamines

Since the use of amphetamines is of questionable value, the taking of these drugs, especially in situations other than those listed under medical treatment, may be considered misuse. The misuse of amphetamines generally revolves around:

1. weight control,
2. increased physical performance, and
3. increased mental performance, alertness, or relief from general lassitude.

Weight control

An exhaustive review of drugs related to obesity has led Pennick to conclude that amphetamines are of limited value in the treatment of obesity [11]. Amphetamines do suppress appetite, but after a while they lose their anorexic effect. Controlled study has shown amphetamines to be of no greater value than placebos in treatment of obesity lasting more than four to eight weeks. The situation in which amphetamines would be of the most value include loss of small amounts of weight (10 to 15 pounds, that which can be safely accomplished in 4 to 8 weeks), control of a sporadic, overwhelming craving for food, or the beginning of a long-term treatment regimen to "set" patterns and add motivation.

Dangers of amphetamine use in relation to weight control include the pattern often referred to as the "housewife syndrome." Along with the "chemical willpower" supplied by amphetamines, they cause an elevation in mood. Gradually, the elevation in mood may become the main reason for taking the diet pill, with the user having a "perfectly good excuse" to take the drug. The user may find that he or she needs that "upper" before starting for work, cleaning the house, or merely facing another day. Then, to avoid depression, another pill or two must be taken during the day. Restlessness and insomnia often result in the increased use of depressants (alcohol, barbiturates, etc.) in the evening and a vicious cycle develops.

Physical performance

We are constantly exposed to reports of drug use among high school, college, and professional athletes [16]. Although probably exaggerated, it has been estimated within the media that 40% of professional athletes use "bennies or greenies." Drug use to increase performance has resulted from a misinterpretation of historical use and scientific study, along with publicity and the basic human desire for achievement. Amphetamines were first used on a large scale during World War II by both sides to keep soldiers, pilots, and factory workers awake when situations demanded that they operate with a minimum of sleep. Early scientific research verified this effect, showing that amphetamines were able to aid performance in certain endeavors. Breaking activity into such components as reaction time, steadiness of the hand, speed, and endurance, and studying each independently and in laboratory conditions has produced inconsistent results, ranging from no improvement in normal subjects to great improvement in subjects fatigued by the lack of sleep for 24 to

60 hours. The majority of laboratory studies conducted in the last ten years show no improvement in speed, strength, or endurance (see the list of suggested reading at the end of this chapter).

It is often difficult to determine whether the activities studied in performance experiments have great significance when compared to actual athletic performance for what is involved in the latter is a complex set of coordinated actions and re actions based on learning, memory, and planning, not to mention the all-important motivation. It makes more sense to test athletes during actual competition, and the numerous "dope testing" programs that have been initiated at various amateur athletic contests such as the Olympics gave researchers that opportunity. Studies of such contests showed greater validity than previous studies because both winners and losers were tested. In Winnipeg in 1967, testing the same number of winners and losers revealed eight athletes who had used amphetamines, of whom three were winners and five were losers. In Rome during the same year it was the cyclists who finished 11, 12, and 14 in a road race who tested positive for amphet amines. In a more recent study it was not until they tested the later finishers that they began to find evidence of drug use; none of the top six finishers had taken drugs, but at least six losers showed evidence of drug use.

Amphetamines act as a stimulant by releasing epinephrine and norepinephrine from the adrenal glands and central nervous system, respectively. The resulting increases in heart rate, blood pressure, glucose and fatty acid levels, accompanied by increased muscle tension and nerve impulses from joints, all bombard the brainstem (more specifically, the reticular activating system). Thus the individual feels more alert, can resist sleep, and experiences less of the general feeling of fa tigue. The athlete interprets these physiological symptoms as an indication of being more "up," more ready to play; thus it is more how one feels than what one does which perpetuates the amphetamine performance myth. Amphetamines produce an elevation in mood, a euphoria, a hyperoptimism which do not allow the performer to realistically evaluate his performance and alter it accordingly. Even in laboratory studies the drugged subject usually cannot believe his or her performance was not better than the results indicated. One former professional football player stated that he had used bennies in only two games and that in both he had been thrown out for overaggressiveness and overzealous rough play. He thought at the time that he was the greatest defensive linebacker ever, but the feeling was subjective, for the grading films showed his many mistakes. In part, his aggressiveness came from getting to the action somewhat slower than usual.

Another problem with the relationship between amphetamines and perfor mance is that of the variability of the drug and the complexities of administration. Dosage, purity, timing, solubility, and tolerance are examples of factors that can alter drug metabolism and an individual's reaction to it, which makes drug usage, at best, a hit-or-miss affair.

One danger of amphetamine use during performance is that of masking fatigue symptoms; this may convince the athlete to perform longer than is safe. When ac companied by heat buildup, the result may be circulatory collapse. Amphetamines tend to make the body less efficient by increasing heart rate and blood pressure beyond what is needed to perform a particular task. Likewise, delays in pulse and respiratory recovery have also been shown. There are numerous examples of deaths among drugged athletes performing such endurance events as long bicycle races.

Mental performance

One of the more widely recognized legitimate uses for amphetamines is to allay the feelings of fatigue and to fight the desire to sleep. As was previously mentioned, amphetamines became popular during World War II for this reason. The Japanese, Germans, British, and Americans gave out millions of energy pills to keep the machinery of war in high gear. Subsequent Army and Air Force studies show that amphetamines enabled soldiers and pilots to function for prolonged periods when drowsiness would have been hazardous. The astronauts used them to fight drowsiness when reentry into the earth's atmosphere happened to take place at the end rather than the beginning of the day.

Although it has been shown that amphetamines will allay the feeling of fatigue and help one fight drowsiness, they have not been shown to increase mental performance in the nonfatigued or rested state. The student needing extra time, the truck driver or salesman fighting the highway hypnosis are making a trade; they are gaining hours, but giving up performance. It has been repeatedly demonstrated that the amphetamine-stimulated mind is able to resist sleep for all-night study sessions, but it is the opinion of most researchers that the fatigued mind (even when stimulated by more amphetamines) cannot learn or reason as well as the unfatigued mind. Furthermore, after the student has managed to stay awake all night, he must either take more of the drug for the testing session or risk the onset of fatigue. Either situation is likely to result in impairment of attention and loss of accuracy, judgment, and problem-solving ability [2]. Just as in the case of the athlete, hyperoptimism does not allow the student to realistically evaluate his performance and alter it accordingly. The student must make a decision based on his particular situation. For students who have not kept up their work during the preceding 15 weeks, the material memorized in an all-night cram session might be worth the decrement in performance during the test. It has been generally concluded that although amphetamines have been shown to enhance a variety of activities, none of the activities reported has been comparable to the experiences faced by the average student [15]. Likewise, truckers and others in similar situations must also realize that the gains in wakefulness and simple reaction time are usually offset by poor judgment and overreaction to stimuli, which often result in highway accidents [2].

THE ABUSE OF AMPHETAMINES AND ITS DANGERS

The term abuse is usually reserved for a pattern of drug use that is viewed as productive of antisocial behavior or as detrimental to the health of the user. Various patterns of amphetamine use have emerged and reemerged over the last 10 years, many of which can be labeled abuse.

One such pattern is a chronic extension or exaggeration of the misuse pattern described in the preceding section. Low-dose oral amphetamines are taken compulsively on a daily basis in a desperate attempt to maintain a stimulated pace of life, to chemically reinforce an outgoing personality, to keep the mood elevated and to hold back the inevitable depression that sets in as the body rebounds from the chronic stimulation. A common pattern usually emerges, uppers in the morning and afternoon, downers such as alcohol and barbiturates at night. In an attempt to reduce some of the nervous side effects of amphetamine stimulation, many commercial brands add sedatives, usually barbiturates, to the amphetamines, resulting in an unintentional barbiturate dependence.

Another pattern of amphetamine abuse lies in the intravenous use of high-dose methamphetamine. Unlike the chronic oral abuse, injected speed use is usually cyclical. Each episode or run may last from several hours to a few days and users are almost always motivated by the extreme euphoric effects [3].

The extreme physical effects of speed are the primary reason for its popularity. Within seconds after feeling the liquid flow into the vein, the user experiences an intense tingling sensation analogous to an electric shock; some appropriately refer to it as a "buzz." This is followed by more intense tingling sensations, some muscle contraction, and an immediate sense of extreme pleasure [10]. It has been hypothesized that this feeling may be the result of rapid release of norepinephrine by amphetamine and subsequent replacement of norepinephrine by a breakdown product of the amphetamine [7]. Numerous reports of orgasms, near-orgasms, and a vibrating feeling of the brain and spinal cord are indicative of intense stimulation of the sympathetic nervous system.

As tolerance develops, initial users progress from doses of around 10–40 mg several times a day to many times that amount as they become chronic users. These amounts are sufficient to activate the thalamus, hypothalamus, and reticular activating system enough to produce prolonged euphoria accompanied by feelings of extreme alertness, increased energy, and clever, insightful, and profound loquaciousness [10]. Users in the group setting profess an ability to relate to the others in frank honesty and with extreme confidence. The excessive conversation is spurred by the belief that what one is saying is profound and that the others desire to listen rather than talk themselves [5, 14].

Amphetamine involvement with the limbic system and the hypothalamus seems to be responsible for many of the effects of speed, including the lack of appetite, insomnia, thirst, and extreme hypersexuality [9]. One who is high on speed exhibits extreme optimism as well as an overextended feeling of love; prolonged body contact with the opposite sex is common, but in most cases expression of love is either forgotten or regretted afterward. This hypersexuality may result, at least in part, from accelerated tactile, auditory, olfactory, and visual impulses [4].

The initial experiences and activities of a speed experience are usually meaningful and purposeful. But as this hyperactive state is prolonged for several hours, he activity becomes progressively more compulsive and disorganized. The period of extreme hyperactivity may last for several days.

Because of amphetamine action on the hypothalamus, extreme anorexia occurs. A large weight loss is not uncommon on long runs. Despite the knowledge that large amounts of vitamins, liquids, and nutritional supplements are necessary, symptoms of malnutrition such as abscesses, ulcers, and brittle fingernails are often observed in speed users. Extreme pain in muscles and joints, accompanied by muscle tremors, often occurs after several days of prolonged use. Serious overdoses are uncommon, but may result in unconsciousness, chest pain, heart throbbing, and a feeling of paralysis [14].

The longer the run persists, the more the scene changes from one of pleasant optimism and euphoria to one of hyperactive aggressiveness; this is not hard to understand, in light of the action of methamphetamine on the limbic and reticular activating systems. Accelerated and intermixed sensory impulses are combined with extreme fatigue caused by sleep deprivation. Unknown tactile, visual, and auditory stimuli appearing in the periphery trigger fear and aggressive responses. This effect is not necessarily inherent in the amphetamine reaction alone, but is a result of group interaction in a situation in which five or six people, hypersensitive to external stimuli, are all moving and talking at once [6]. Psychoticlike characteristics begin to appear. Objects are observed in detail and the individual becomes overly concerned with attaching significance to even inanimate objects such as cracks in the wall, dirt, etc. These are often mistaken for micro-animals and snakes, and adverse emotional reactions may occur. Also common to amphetamine psychosis is an inability to recognize faces, which leads to suspiciousness and a feeling of being watched. This paranoia often results in an acute psychotic reaction [13].

Much has been written on the aggressiveness and violence associated with the speed scene. It should be repeated that this violence is the result of an excessively long run, and is especially likely to occur when all available speed has been used. The fatigued and irritated user then goes out in search of more speed or a place to crash. Both situations create an environment that can easily trigger the potential hostility.

Likewise, the extreme irritability of the speed user during the post-high depression makes finding a place to crash a problem. Friends, even those who use speed, do not want to expose themselves to an argumentative, potentially violent individual who is likely to attack with little provocation. This situation serves to augment the depression of the crash, which is so profound and intense that shooting up again is almost a necessity.

Paranoia and violence

Intravenous, high-dose amphetamine inevitably leads to some degree of paranoia and the wise user can prepare for it. But, as was described in the preceding section, long and intense runs usually result in a loss of rationality and as time goes on, the hypersensitivity, visual and tactile illusions, and fatigue state may cause paranoia.

Once the user experiences extreme paranoia, a return to the same level of conscious ness often triggers a similar experience. Extreme hyperactivity, fatigue, paranoia, an the social condition are all responsible for the increased violence associated wit high-dose amphetamine use. The user changes moods rapidly and is irrational in th evaluation of a situation; thus coping behavior is overreactive and aggressive [8].

Psychosis

Most psychoactive drugs have the ability to trigger a psychotic episode in psychosis prone individuals, but study of chronic amphetamine users suggests that psychosi is not idiosyncratic, but an inevitable consequence of chronic high-dose amphet amine abuse. Acute psychotic episodes can be precipitated by an exaggeration o many of the conditions normally found in the amphetamine experience, i.e., lack c sleep, visual and tactile illusions, visual and auditory hallucinations, lack of food extreme anxiety, paranoid delusions, aggressiveness, and irritability. Psychosis re lated to amphetamine abuse is acute and may reoccur with additional use, but usu ally is not chronic and does not carry over into the nondrug state unless the indi vidual is psychotic-prone [10].

Overdoses and death

Amphetamine overdoses, more often called "over-amping" (a term derived from th use of too many ampules containing liquid methamphetamine), are uncommon anc not fatal. A user can develop a tolerance to the awakening effects of the drug, whicl often leads to use of amounts hundreds of times the clinical dose. Symptoms such a: extreme chest pain, unconsciousness, aphasia, mental and/or physical paralysis, anc erratically racing thought patterns often lead to shooting up again and hence ar exaggeration of the problem that may require hospitalization.

Death is more often caused by chronic toxicity of amphetamines or by socia conditions surrounding the user. Viral hepatitis is not an uncommon conditior among those who share unsterilized hypodermic equipment. Hepatic damage as a direct toxic effect of amphetamines has also been suggested. If not properly carec for, infection from skin lesions and endocarditis may also cause death in extreme cases.

OTHER STIMULANTS

Other stimulants that deserve mention are cocaine, nicotine, and caffeine. The stimu latory effects of nicotine will be discussed further in the chapter on smoking, but it should be mentioned that nicotine causes a mood elevation that is usually interpreted as having a calming effect or a control of excess nervousness, restlessness, and irrita bility. The effect is mild when compared to amphetamine and cocaine, but cigarettes are usually used constantly throughout the day. The absence of a cigarette in a chronic smoker results in a slight depression from the normal nicotine-elevated mood and offers continual motivation to "light up."

Caffeine is the stimulant found in coffee, tea, and soft drinks labeled cola or pepper. The stimulating effects of caffeine are mild when compared to those of amphetamines, but to a lesser extent they produce the same reaction, namely liberation of epinephrine which results in slight increases in heart rate, blood pressure, and may cause muscle tremors, restlessness, and insomnia. As with nicotine cigarettes, caffeine drinks can be consumed regularly throughout the day, thus allowing for a continuous mood elevation. Caffeine pills have become popular as antifatigue agents; they are sold over the counter and are often passed off as amphetamines on the illegal market.

Cocaine

Cocaine is a powerful central nervous system stimulant derived from the leaves of the *Erythroxylon coca* plant native to South America. Natives of Peru and Bolivia have chewed coca leaves for centuries, primarily to alleviate hunger and fatigue from strenuous work at high altitudes. Cocaine has been praised and damned throughout the years and its popularity has likewise increased and decreased. Cocaine was used in the practice of medicine by such notables as Sigmund Freud, who experimented with it personally and recommended it to his patients. Noting the relief of not only depression but also many of the physical symptoms that bothered his patients, Freud considered it a wonder drug until he observed its dependence-producing potential. Cocaine was also used as a local anesthetic by plastic surgeons and was an ingredient in popular drinks like Coca-Cola in the late 1800s.

The popularity of cocaine diminished in the years after passage of the Harrison Narcotic Act of 1914. Confiscation at border checkpoints and medical reports in the late 1960s signalled an increase in cocaine use, and by 1972 cocaine popularity had increased several-fold. The reasons for the sudden increase in popularity are not known, but some have hypothesized that publicity created a snowball effect. Another factor may be the development in recent years of the interior Amazon region, creating accessibility to greater amounts of cocaine, along with the establishment of sophisticated smuggling organizations. Like heroin, cocaine is expensive on the street and yields a good profit to those willing to take the risks of selling it. As with other drugs sold illegally without regulation or quality control, cocaine is adulterated, being cut with cheap synthetics such as Procaine, Benzocaine, and speed.

In pure form cocaine is a white crystalline powder (sometimes called "snow"), and is either sniffed in powder form or liquefied and subsequently injected. It appears that the latter method is currently preferred because cocaine sniffing involves the physical complication of deterioration of the lining of nasal passageways and, eventually, of the nasal septum. Often cocaine is mixed with heroin so that the stimulatory effects will not be so intense, and it is found that many cocaine users use heroin or some other depressant to tide them over between cocaine binges, only to find that they have become physically dependent on the depressant.

Because cocaine is short-acting, it may be used repeatedly, and excessive amounts (up to 10 grams) may be taken within a single day. A lethal dose is approximately 1200 milligrams for most individuals, if the entire amount is taken at once. Death is due to respiratory failure.

The reason for repeated use of cocaine is much like that for methamphetamine —the user ascends to extreme heights of mood elevation, elation, and grandiosity. When this feeling begins to wane, depression sets in, and another dose of cocaine is strongly desired. (No physical dependence is involved, nor does tolerance develop.) Continued use results in loss of appetite, loss of weight, malnutrition, insomnia, digestive disorders, paranoia, and hallucinations, especially tactile hallucinations known as "the cocaine bugs." Much like the speed freak, the chronic cocaine user becomes socially dangerous because of the mental aberrations caused by his or her drug [12].

REFERENCES

1. Alles, G. A., "The Comparative Physiological Action of Phenylethanolamine," *Journal of Pharmacology and Experimental Therapy*, 32:121–133, 1927.

2. AMA Committee on Alcoholism and Addiction and Council on Mental Health, "Dependence on Amphetamines and Other Stimulants," *Journal of the American Medical Association*, 197:1023–1028, 1966.

3. Cohen, S., "Amphetamine Abuse," *Journal of the American Medical Association*, 231:414–415, 1975.

4. Ellinwood, E. H., "Amphetamine Psychosis II. Theoretical Implications," *International Journal of Neuropsychiatry*, 4:45–54, 1968.

5. Ellinwood, E. H., and M. M. Kilbey, "Amphetamine Stereotypy," *Biological Psychiatry*, 10(1):3–16, 1975.

6. Fischer, C. M., *et al.*, "Behavioral Mediators in the Polyphasic Mortality Curve of Aggregate Amphetamine Toxicity," *Journal of Psychedelic Drugs*, 2:55–62, 1970.

7. Griffith, J. D., *et al.*, "Schizophreniform Psychosis Induced by Large-Dose Administration of d-Amphetamine," *Journal of Psychedelic Drugs*, 2:42–48, 1970.

8. Grinspoon, L., and P. Hedblom, *The Speed Culture: Amphetamine Use in America.* Cambridge, Mass.: Harvard Press, 1975.

9. Idanpaan-Heikkila, J. E., *et al.*, "Relation of Pharmacological and Behavioral Effects of a Hallucinogenic Amphetamine to Distribution in Cat Brain," *Science*, 196:1085–1086, 1969.

10. Kramer, J. C., *et al.*, "Amphetamine Abuse," *Journal of the American Medical Association*, 210:305–309, 1967.

11. Pennick, S. B., "Amphetamines in Obesity," *Seminars in Psychiatry*, 1:144, 1969.

12. Post, R. M., "Cocaine Psychosis: A Continuum Model," *American Journal of Psychiatry*, 132(3):225–231, 1975.

13. Smith, D. E., "The Psychotomimetic Amphetamines with Special Reference to STP (DOM) Toxicity," *Journal of Psychedelic Drugs*, 2:73–85, 1970.

14. Smith, R. C., and D. Crim, "The World of the Haight-Ashbury Speed Freak," *Journal of Psychedelic Drugs*, 2:172–188, 1970.

15. Smith, S. M., and P. H. Blanchy, "Amphetamine Usage by Medical Students," *Journal of Medical Education,* 41:167–171, 1966.

16. Wrighton, J. D., "Doping in Sport," *Nursing Times,* 71(1):35–36, 1975.

SUGGESTED READING

"Amphetamine-Type Drugs for Hyperactive Children," *Medical Letter on Drugs and Therapeutics,* 14:21–23, 1972.

Breitner, C., "Appetite-Suppressing Drugs as an Etilogic Factor and Mental Illness," *Psychosomatics,* 4:327–333, 1963.

Caldwell, J., *et al.,* "The Biochemical Pharmacology of Abused Drugs I. Amphetamines, Cocaine, LSD," *Clinical Pharmacology and Therapeutics,* 16(4):625–638, 1974.

Cameron, J. S., *et al.,* "Effects of Amphetamines on Moods, Emotions and Motivations," *Journal of Psychology,* 61:93–121, 1965.

Connell, P. H., *Amphetamine Psychosis.* London: Chapman and Hall, 1958.

Connell, P. H., "Clinical Manifestations and Treatment of Amphetamine Type of Dependence," *Journal of the American Medical Association,* 196:718–723, 1966.

Edwards, R. E., "Abuse of Central Nervous System Stimulants," *American Journal of Hospital Pharmacy,* 22:145–148, 1965.

Ellinwood, E. H., and S. Cohen, "Amphetamine Abuse," *Science,* 171:420–421, 1971.

Geissmann, P., and C. Geissmann, "A Study of Depression Following the Taking of Appetite Killers," *Bordeaux Medical,* 2:115–119, 1972.

Gilbert, B., "Drugs in Sports," *Sports Illustrated,* June 23, June 30, July 7, 1969.

Green, M. H., *et al.,* "Amphetamines in the District of Columbia III," *International Journal of the Addictions,* 9(5):652–662, 1974.

Guldberg, H. C., and C. A. Marsden, "Brain Monoamines and the Increase in Motor Activity in the Rate after Amphetamine," *British Journal of Pharmacology,* 44:347P–48P, 1972.

Hawks, David, "Abuse of Methylamphetamine," *British Medical Journal,* 2:915–920, 1969.

Kalant, H., *et al.,* "Death in Amphetamine Users; Causes and Rates," *Canadian Medical Association Journal,* 112(3):299–304, 1975.

Kavaler, L., *The Amphetamines.* Springfield, Ill.: Charles C. Thomas, 1966.

Kosman, Mary E., "Effects of Chronic Administration of the Amphetamines and Other Stimulants on Behavior," *Clinical Pharmacology and Therapeutics,* 9:240–254, 1968.

Kramer, J. C., *et al.,* "Amphetamine Abuse: Pattern and Effects of High Doses Taken intravenously," *Journal of the American Medical Association,* 197:1023, 1966.

Lemere, F., "The Danger of Amphetamine Dependency," *American Journal of Psychiatry,* 123:5, 1966.

Louria, Donald B., *Nightmare Drugs.* New York: Pocket Books, 1966.

McCormick, T. C., Jr., "Toxic Reaction to Amphetamines," *Diseases of the Nervous System,* 23:219–224, 1962.

Morgan, Diana, *et al.*, "Amphetamine Analogues and Brain Amines," *Life Sciences* 11:83–96, 1972.

Offermeier, J., and B. Potgieter, "The Possible Central Stimulant Mechanisms of Some Appetite Suppressants," *South African Medical Journal*, 46:72–77, 1972.

Pierson, W. R., "Amphetamine Sulfate and Performance (a Critique)," *Journal of the American Medical Association*, 177(5):345–349, 1971.

"Psychotropic Agents and the Hyperkinetic," *Medical World News*, 13:60, 1972.

Salsbury, C. A., *et al.*, "The Uses and Misuses of Amphetamines," *Medicolegal Bulletin* 156:1–9, 1966.

Scott, P. D., "Delinquency and the Amphetamines," *British Journal of Psychiatry*, 111: 865–875, 1965.

Sussman, Sidney, "Narcotic and Methamphetamine Use During Pregnancy: Effect on Newborn Infants," *American Journal Diseases of Children*, 106:125–130, 1963.

TERMINOLOGY OF AMPHETAMINES AND OTHER STIMULANTS

All lit up	Under the influence of a drug
Amine	A substance having an NH_2 group in its chemical structure
Antidepressant	A chemical that counteracts depressed feelings
Bang	Inject, or get a thrill from injection
Benny	Benzedrine, an amphetamine
Benny jag	High on Benzedrine
Black beauties	Biphetamine
Blue velvet	A paregoric antihistamine mixture
C	Cocaine
Cartwheels	Amphetamine tablets scored into quarters
Christmas trees	Dexamyl
Coke	Cocaine
Coming down	Coming off a drug high
Co-pilots	Amphetamines
Crash	Come down from a prolonged high
Crystal	Methamphetamine
Dexie	Dexedrine
Drivers, or truckdrivers	Amphetamines
Dynamite	High-grade heroin, sometimes mixed with cocaine
Euphoria	An exaggerated sense of well-being
Eye openers	Amphetamines
Factory	Place for the manufacture of illicit drugs
Fives	5-milligram tablets, usually amphetamines
Flake	Cocaine

Flash	A sudden rush of euphoria after injection of methamphetamine or heroin
Freakout	A bad experience, or temporary psychotic reaction
Fruit salad	A game of taking many different pills
Glow	High, euphoriant
Hallucinations	Perceptions with no external reality
Hearts	Amphetamine tablets so shaped
Jolly beans	Pep pills
Joy-pop or skin-pop	Inject drugs under the skin
Mainline	Inject drugs into a vein
Meth	Methamphetamine
On	Under the influence of drugs
Oranges	Dexedrine tablets
O.T.C.	Over-the-counter drugs, sold without prescription
Peachies	Benzedrine in tablet form
Paper	Paper for writing prescriptions
Pep pills	Amphetamines
Pillhead	Person using amphetamines or barbiturates in pill form
Pop	Take drugs orally or inject them under the skin
Rush	Sudden onset of euphoria
Shoot up	Inject drugs
Shooting gallery	A safe place to shoot up
Snow	Cocaine
Speed	Methamphetamine
Speed freak	Habitual user of speed
Square	Nonuser
Stoned	High on drugs
Street, on the street	Out searching for drugs
Strung out	Caught up in drug use
Tingle	Rush or high feeling
Uppers	Stimulants
Wired	High on drugs, especially amphetamines
Yen	Strong desire for drugs

7 SMOKING AND HEALTH

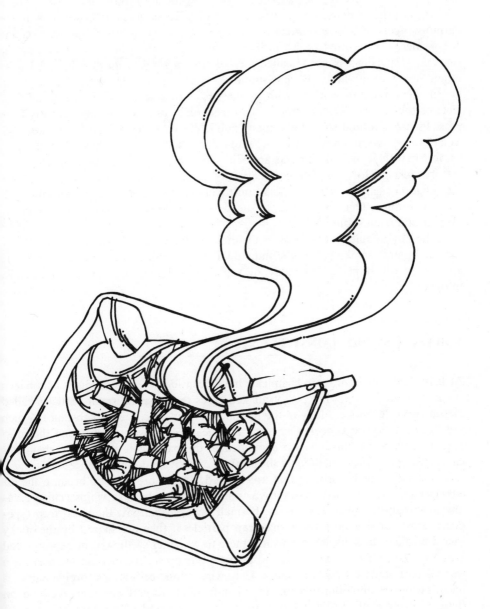

Next to caffeine, nicotine is the most widely used stimulant, even though it has been well documented that smoking contributes generously to the national morbidity and mortality rates. Nevertheless, apparently 40% of the adult population have chosen to disregard the evidence and continue to smoke. To subject one's own body to the harmful effects of tobacco smoke is usually regarded as an individual decision and is considered a personal health problem. But not all the smoke is inhaled by the smoker. That which is not is called the sidestream smoke and may be inhaled by others in close proximity. Recent studies [14, 15, 28, 29, 31] have indicated that nonsmokers living or working with smokers likewise suffer some of the harmful effects of tobacco smoke. To protect the nonsmoker, ordinances have recently been passed which prohibit smoking in many public places, especially enclosed ones such as elevators, and in many cities it is "smokers to the back of the bus!" While smokers feel that their individual rights are being violated, groups representing nonsmokers are pushing for complete eradication of public smoking. Thus, even smoking the tobacco cigarette has become a controversial issue which has philosophical or moral overtones. One may choose to smoke, but does one have the right to alter the air that others must breathe?

The physiological consequences of smoking, the psychological and social forces for and against smoking, and the individual rights versus public safety controversy are issues which make the study of smoking and smoking behavior especially intriguing.

TOBACCO SMOKE CONSTITUENTS

At least 1200 different toxic chemicals have been identified as products of tobacco smoke. Smoke is a mixture of hot air and gases that suspend small particles called *tars* in cigarette smoke. Many of the particles contain *carcinogens,* substances which are known to cause cancer. One such chemical, benzopyrene, is among the most potent carcinogens known. Also contained in the particulate matter are chemicals called *phenols,* which are thought to speed up or activate dormant cancer cells.

Normally, small particles that are inhaled are not problematic because the air passageways are cleansed constantly as millions of tiny hairlike whips (cilia) escalate mucus up the respiratory tract. If small particles get past the nasal trap (specially constructed wind tunnels that trap particles), they are snared by the sticky mucal escalator and are taken upward, there to be either swallowed or expectorated (see Fig. 7.1). If particles happen to get past this protective mechanism, there is a third line of defense within the lungs. Here white blood cells attack foreign particles and destroy or immobilize them. In an individual without constant overload on these protective devices, the lungs are normally cleared of dangerous materials. However, if a smoker constantly overloads this system, or if an individual works amid coal dust or other constantly inhaled particles, or if a person lives in an air-polluted environment, this system cannot remove particles effectively and there is danger of deleterious effects. Then as cigarette tar is deposited on normal respira-

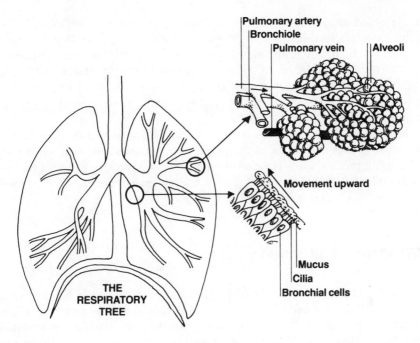

Figure 7.1

ory tract cells, some chemicals in the smoke irritate the cells, some bring about the ancer process, and still others speed up this process.

Aiding the tars in their deleterious effects on the respiratory system is the action f various *gases* within cigarette smoke. The gases of importance here are ammonia, ormaldehyde, acetaldehyde, and hydrogen cyanide (a strong poison in itself). These our gases combine to immobilize the cilia of the air passageways for six to eight ours, and it is obvious what happens to the "mucus escalator" when the ciliary novement ceases. No longer can particles be normally removed; hence, when they nter the respiratory tract, they can directly affect the mucus-producing and ciliary ells. It is as though two protective coverings have been removed and the underlying ells laid bare to the irritation of cigarette tars. Some of the cilia-producing and nucus-producing cells, then, are completely destroyed over a period of time. In an ccasional smoker (e.g., one who smokes a pack or less a week) there may be sufcient time after each cigarette for the cilia to recover; however, a heavy smoker (a ack or more a day) rarely allows this recovery time and permanent damage occurs. he absence of the cilia-mucus protective coating and clearing device makes the smoker's cough" a necessity to clear phlegm, or particles large enough to affect the oughing mechanism, from the air passageways. The damage to these cells of the espiratory tract also makes the smoker more susceptible to upper respiratory infecons and chronic bronchitis.

Another constituent of tobacco smoke is *nicotine,* the drug component. Nicotine a stimulant of the central nervous system which, like others in this class, produces distinct physiological and psychological changes in the human organism. Nicotir does not cause physical dependence, but a tolerance to its effects does develop. Th stimulation or high can result in a psychological dependence that may be a sig nificant factor in habituation to cigarette smoking. Nicotine effects on the cardi< vascular system are responsible for the strong statistical link between cigarette smol ing and diseases of the cardiovascular system and will be considered in more deta later in this chapter.

The amount of tar and nicotine in tobacco is determined by such factors a plant strain, processing, origin of the plant, growth conditions, heat and humidit and the aging process used. How much of the tar and nicotine gets into the syste depends on how the tobacco is used: whether it is chewed, taken as snuff, or smoke< and, of course, whether it is inhaled or not.

MOTIVATIONS FOR SMOKING

Most people start smoking for social reasons and continue out of habit or satisfa< tion of a psychological need. Statistics reveal that most heavy smokers take up th habit before the age of 20. Statistics vary, but over the last four years smokin among high school (grades 9–12) students has increased anywhere from four 1 eight percent. One recent study found as many as 41% of males and 39% of f< males in the twelfth grade to be regular smokers. Another trend emerging is that < equality of the sexes, as women approach an equal position in the male-dominate smoking statistics [13].

A logical question at this point is, why doesn't someone tell the teenage popula tion that smoking is a dangerous habit? Recent studies suggest that they alread know. McRae and Nelson [20] found that 83.3% of smokers and 96.2% of nor smokers considered smoking hazardous to one's health. Other studies show similarl high percentages—90% [1] and 96.7% [18]—of enlightened teenagers. If they po: sess this knowledge, why the increase in smoking among teenagers? Why the utt< disregard for their health?

It is becoming increasingly obvious that teenagers have not incorporated th maintenance of health into their intrinsic value system. It is difficult for them t imagine any upset of that ever-present flow of energy and strength that abound within them. The teenage years are not usually directed by inner motivations, bt are more often directed by peer influence. This is an important observation, for smol ing is, at least in the initial stage of the habit, a sociological phenomenon. Man people need oral gratification, but mainly those who have been oriented to smokin by family and/or friends will accept it as part of their lives. Research helps sul stantiate this by showing that ninth-graders exhibit smoking behavior identical 1 that of their best friends [24], and that children have a 50% greater chance < starting smoking if their parents smoke [10]. As students progress through hig school and the sanctions against smoking are lessened, friendships among smoke) and nonsmokers become commonplace. Even though high schoolers are better abl accept individual differences and are more internally motivated, parents, teachers, siblings, and peers still influence many to start smoking. Likewise, one cannot disregard smoking as a symbol of independence or of being grown-up.

The sudden disappearance of these motivators would still leave a very forceful one—that of advertising. Even without television advertising, cigarette manufacturers spend more than 300 million dollars each year not only promoting one particular brand over another, but generally promoting the acceptance of smoking. A closer look at cigarette advertising clearly shows that very few facts about the cigarette are presented. The words are rather trite and meaningless, for few take the time to read them. The ads draw on the individual needs and memory of good feeling by presenting a picture of a pleasant and happy situation. Because there exists a universal need for love or at least companionship, and a desire for escape and adventure, the scene portrays an attractive couple obviously in love and enjoying themselves, or shows the rugged man out in the wilds of nature or the woman taking a much deserved minute of relaxation. The ads are designed to reduce one's anxieties about growing old, losing one's health, being alone, or losing sex drive. Or they may attempt to appeal to one's ego, by implying that they have something more than the other guy. The impact of such advertising on potential smokers is substantial and it has been shown that sales are directly related to capital expenditure for advertising. Most smokers cannot even distinguish their favorite brand when blindfolded, which makes a "taste" factor highly questionable in choice of brand. A particular brand is chosen because of identification with the feeling portrayed by the advertisement or perhaps identification with someone who also smokes that particular brand.

But still the cigarette must deliver. Smoking must satisfy a need of the smoker or smoking behavior would be extinguished. As previously mentioned, nicotine is a mild stimulant; thus a slight elevation in mood often results. This is usually interpreted as relaxation, a feeling of ease, of being in control of one's "nervous energy." But usually it goes deeper than that. Smoking is abuse of a chemical substance and an abuse of oral gratification, and it usually develops into a habit. Although theories on the deeper psychological motivations are not well developed, studies on teenage smokers suggest a relationship between the need to smoke and feelings of insecurity and low self-esteem.

As we have seen in print so many times, adolescence is a confusing and trying time. Teenagers often demand so much of themselves that success and satisfaction are nearly impossible. Smoking has been called a psychological compensatory action, engaged in by those who experience failure. Although failure to meet one's internal expectations is difficult to measure, it often results in low self-esteem, which has been observed more in smoking teenagers than in nonsmoking ones. Since failure often results in diversion of efforts from assigned tasks, it is little wonder that teenage smokers seem to experience more failure in school than do nonsmokers [25]. Newman [23] has found that smokers generally perceive themselves as not meeting the expectations of their parents. This perception gives rise to a certain amount of alienation, and it is little wonder that teenage smokers are more apt to give "nonestablishment" responses to questionnaires. It has also been found that teenage smokers tend to get lower grades, create more discipline problems, and participate

less in school activities than do their nonsmoking counterparts. Placed in a sociolog
cal milieu in which smoking is acceptable (in the teenage world, often encouraged)
smoking often becomes an unconscious attempt to gain satisfaction.

In the late 1950s and early 1960s several studies correlating smoking wit
specific psychological and behavioral characteristics were reported: the smoker wa
characterized as being more restless, nervous, extroverted, energetic, thrill-seekin
independent, etc.; while nonsmokers were characterized as puritanical, conservative
stable, agreeable, dependable, religious, etc. The male smoker was reportedly les
masculine and made a poorer prospect for marriage and employment. Heavy con
sumers of tobacco were also shown to be the heaviest consumers of alcohol, coffee
and candy [26].

The personality differences between smokers and nonsmokers that have bee
found tell only part of the story. Believing that the smoker's personality is drug
prone and pathological would lead one to the conclusion that nearly one-half of th
adult American population is maladjusted or abnormal. Maladjusted perhaps, bu
that high a percentage of people cannot be abnormal. It might be more enlightenin
to view the difference between smokers and nonsmokers in the following manner
The smoker probably grew up in an environment in which family and/or peer
encouraged smoking; thus he or she learned to smoke to satisfy needs. The non
smoker probably grew up in an environment in which family and peers discourage
smoking; thus he or she learned to satisfy needs with other compensatory activities
or perhaps had fewer needs to be satisfied.

There is no one characteristic, one abnormality, one need, one insecurity tha
leads to smoking, for even within the ranks of smokers, at least four different type
of smokers have been identified. Which type are you?

1. Do you smoke more in times of crisis? Have you frequently quit smoking, bu
seemed to lapse back into smoking behavior during particularly stressful times? Doe
your cigarette seem to be a sedative, reducing negative feelings of fear, anger, o
nervousness? If so, you can be classified as a *negative-effect smoker,* one who uses
cigarette as a crutch in times of crisis or as a sedative to relieve negative feeling
such as nervousness, anger, shame, or disgust. This kind of need fulfillment offer
tremendous reinforcement and smoking becomes a very pleasurable experience.

2. Do you find yourself lighting one cigarette before the other is completely out?
Does the lack of a cigarette create an uncomfortable feeling? Do you constantly fee
a strong desire to smoke? Then the chances are that you are an *addictive smoker*
one who uses cigarettes to satisfy needs or to solve problems, one who feels more
normal with a cigarette than without one.

3. Do you really like to smoke and enjoy the taste of smoke? Does smoking relax
you? Does it add enjoyment to a meal? Do you get pleasure from manipulating the
cigarette, blowing smoke rings? Do you think you look older and more sophisti
cated when you smoke? If so, the chances are that you are a *positive-effect smoker*
often called a pleasure smoker.

4. If you are constantly running out of cigarettes, it is likely that you underestimate
the amount you smoke. You are a chain smoker, but it is so automatic that the

igarette is out of the pack and into your mouth almost without conscious thought. 'ou may find that cigarettes don't taste particularly good, but you seem to have one t at all times. Often you light one up only to find one lit in the ashtray. If this be- avior describes your smoking pattern, then what you have is a habit. The *habitual moker* is an "automatic cigarette lighter-upper."

;IVING UP THE HABIT

)ne of the first steps in giving up smoking is to establish what type of smoker you re, since different cessation programs are designed for different types of smokers. If ou cannot answer some of the questions listed above, then begin by observing your moking behavior. You might attach a small note card to your cigarette pack with a rubber band. Every time you take one out, note on the card the time of day, the ctivity you are engaged in, the feeling or mood you are in, perhaps even the com-)any you are in. At the very least, you will find out how many cigarettes you smoke luring a day and whether there is an association with moods, activities, or particular riends. If this progresses satisfactorily, you may even begin analyzing what there is about a particular activity or friend that makes you desire a cigarette.

From this the smoker can select one of the numerous cessation ideas or pro- grams most likely to be of value. First and foremost is motivation—one cannot be 'orced to stop. There must be an intrinsic reason. Most often it is health, but health alone may not be enough reason to invest the time and energy required to break a trong habit. Often it is the desire to show that one still has self-control. Every now and then one may become aware that he or she is eating too much, loafing around, vatching too much television, or smoking too much. To lose weight, to get back into shape, to finish some delayed project, or to quit smoking shows self-control and enhances self-concept and self-respect. Also, with the price of cigarettes constantly ncreasing, to quit smoking may save several hundred dollars in one year's time [4].

Once convinced that smoking is not for you and once armed with some knowl- edge of the reason for your smoking, you may wish to join an organized cessation plan or attempt to quit on your own. If you decide on the latter, choose a method that best fits your smoking behavior. (For example, the habitual smoker can usu- ally obtain success by tapering off.) Concentrate on one situation at a time. Stop smoking when you talk on the telephone, and then stop having one with your coffee. Develop the habit of consciously not having a cigarette with each activity and eventually you will become a habitual nonsmoker [27].

If you are a positive-effect or pleasure smoker, again a tapering-off method might work for you. Use substitutes; switch to cigars or to a pipe. Find something else to manipulate with your hands. Identify the one or two times a day when you obtain the most pleasure from a cigarette and smoke only during those times. Sta- tistics show that people who smoke fewer than five cigarettes per day are only slightly worse off, in terms of health, than the nonsmoker.

If you are a negative-effect smoker, your task is much more difficult. If the act

of smoking relieves anxiety, to stop smoking might create more anxiety. The substitution of eating to relieve anxiety, while not as physically harmful as smoking, is a
poor crutch. In this case a deeper look at one's life-style must be taken in order to
identify and reduce the situations that cause the anxiety. The "cold-turkey" technique is usually best in this situation, as are aversion and deconditioning techniques.

For the person who is an addictive smoker the task is most difficult of all. This
person may need to merely take some of the health hazards out of smoking. He or
she might switch to a low tar and nicotine brand, cut down on the number of puffs
per cigarette, or smoke only half of the cigarette. Perhaps this smoker can even
learn not to inhale or to inhale less deeply.

Negative-effect and addictive smokers usually benefit most from the organized
programs listed below:

1. Lobeline and other nicotine substances. Clinics offering this method provide
literature, lectures, and self-behavior analysis, and substitute medication such as
lobeline (a nicotine substitute given by injection or lobeline sulfate tablets available
without a prescription), together with counseling. Treatment periods vary from a
week to several months.

2. The Five-Day Plan. In five (usually evening) sessions of 90 to 120 minutes
lectures, group discussions, and inspirational, motivating AA-type speeches are presented. Often special diets and activities are recommended, such as daily physical
exercise, walking after meals, heavy consumption of fluid, and liberal use of fruits
and fruit juices. Group discussions on social engineering techniques, such as recognizing and avoiding unnecessary tension or friends who cause anxiety, are a very
important part of the program, as is establishing the buddy system to help control
the urge to smoke. The Seventh Day Adventists have been sponsoring such programs for years, but many other groups also use the plan.

3. Conditioning techniques. This is a clinical approach based on the stimulus-
response learning theory. Smoking becomes associated with unpleasant feelings
through psychotherapy, hypnosis, or some other long-established aversion therapy
technique. Nonsmoking is associated with pleasant feelings and is positively reinforced. The goal is usually a reduction in the number of cigarettes smoked, rather
than complete cessation.

4. Group discussion and therapy techniques. These are the direct opposite of conditioning programs. They deal with the causes of smoking, analyzing one's motivations and talking out problems that lead to the desire to smoke. Group therapy using
sensitivity training, group dynamics, and group pressure helps to reinforce nonsmoking behavior. Participants are urged to quit cold turkey. Jacobs *et al.* [16] suggest
that individuals quitting abruptly see themselves as nonsmokers and reinforce this
perception during group sessions. They also enjoy a special status in the group and
their pride reinforces their self-esteem. The more group members who publicly proclaim their success, the more determined each one becomes to remain abstinent. The
increase in self-esteem, the feeling of accomplishment, and the feeling of self-
mastery become positive reinforcers. Most of the group methods are of multidimen-

onal approach, combining counseling, medication, and education with role-playing nd group discussions [19].

The role of one's personal physician is also very important. The physician can rovide the initial incentive to quit smoking, suggest techniques of cessation, and ct as a counselor. Perhaps most important, the physician can bring to the attention f the smoker the overwhelming evidence concerning the health consequences of moking, which are presented in the remainder of this chapter.

THE HEALTH CONSEQUENCES OF SMOKING

Heart disease

Most of the excess deaths among smokers (deaths beyond the number encountered among nonsmokers) are due to the *drug effects of nicotine* on the circulatory system, which lead to heart disease. Coronary artery disease accounts for about 45% of the total excess deaths related to smoking; then, if one adds the excess deaths from other heart diseases, general arteriosclerosis and hypertensive heart disease, the total of preventable deaths associated with heart disease accounts for more than 50% of all excess deaths in smokers [5].

Nicotine, as a stimulant, affects the human system in a manner similar to that of the amphetamines; that is, it increases heart rate and blood pressure, and other changes occur that are normally attributed to the sympathetic nervous system. However, nicotine works in a two-fold manner to stimulate the system. First, it directly affects cholinergic nerve synapses by mimicking acetylcholine. This not only elicits greater excitability, but also blocks out meaningful impulses that would normally be directed by acetylcholine. After initially exciting these nerve fibers, nicotine "overloads" the ability of the nerve cells to respond, and a blocking effect takes place at the synapse [2, 7].

The second way in which nicotine affects the nervous system is through its action on the adrenal glands. It causes these endocrines to release adrenal hormones, which circulate in the blood, causing excitation of the sympathetic nervous system. In addition to exciting the adrenals, nicotine releases these same hormones from other sites as well, thus completing its sympathomimetic action [11].

When a smoker takes nicotine into his lungs, the substance is quickly taken up by the blood and carried to all parts of the body. Then all these excitatory effects caused by nicotine combine to overwork the heart. If a smoker's heart is exposed to these events 10, 20, or more times a day (often in rapid succession), it will almost certainly be adversely affected.

Nicotine is also thought to be responsible for the elevated plasma-free fatty acids found in smokers. The exact physiological mechanism has not been determined, but sympathetic nervous system and adrenocortical stimulation is known to be activated by nicotine, and must play an important role in the release of fatty acids from adipose deposits.

The carbon monoxide in the gaseous phase of cigarette smoke is thought to significantly decrease cardiac work capacity. Hemoglobin picks up the carbon monoxide from the lungs forming carboxyhemoglobin, which alters myocardial metabolism, interferes with oxygen delivery, and results in myocardial hypoxia [6].

One significant trend that has been taking shape in recent years is the increase in sudden death from coronary heart disease in female smokers. A study of autopsy populations showed that the male-to-female mortality ratio for nonsmokers was 11:1 and it was 3.8:1 for smokers [30].

In summary, we can say that cigarette smoking is related to cardiovascular disease in the following areas:

1. Increased heart rate

2. Increased peripheral vasoconstriction, which in turn causes increased blood pressure

3. Release of fatty acids from adipose stores, thus elevating the level of circulating fats, which are known precursors of atherosclerotic plaques

4. Reduction of blood clotting time

5. Reduction of the amount of oxygen delivered to the tissues by the carbon monoxide content of smoke.

Lung cancer

Serious chronic health problems other than heart disease that are related to cigarette smoking are due mainly to the particulate and gaseous contents of smoke, rather than the sympathomimetic action of nicotine.

The second major cause of excess deaths due to smoking is cancer, most of that being lung cancer. Lung cancer started to become increasingly apparent in the 1920s and 1930s and has grown into a full-blown epidemic since that time. This outbreak of lung cancer not so curiously followed the sharp rise in cigarette use in the United States during World War I—and it followed it by approximately 20 years, the average time involved in producing cancer. To support this temporal theory of lung cancer it was found that Iceland produced the same pattern with a sharp rise in cigarette consumption during World War II, followed by a lung cancer "epidemic" about 20 years later. In 1974 approximately 40,000 people died of lung cancer in the United States, and for middle-aged men, cancer represents the second leading cause of death.

As is well documented now, cigarette tars or particulate matter (the particles enabling one to see smoke) that come into constant contact with the respiratory tract cause a slow change in cells of that system. In time this change may cause the cell to reproduce a cell that is a modification of the original productive one. New cells without productive function are cancer cells—they multiply rapidly and compete with normal cells for nutrients, slowly killing off and replacing normal cells, and normal function of the system is affected.

Carcinoma of the bronchi accounts for approximately 95% of the malignant tumors found in the lung. Both lungs have an equal chance of being affected. About

5% of the bronchial tumors arise from the main stem or first bronchi division, the
section that is the first to be exposed as the smoke enters the lungs. At this point the
smoke is at its fullest concentration, but particles smaller than 0.4 microns will settle
out and become deposited, especially on ridges and bifurcations, just as the sediment
in a river forms a delta.

Bronchogenic carcinomas can be subclassified on the basis of cell histology. The
most predominant (60% of the total) is the epidermoid or squamous cell carcinoma
which, incidentally, is virtually always associated with cigarette smoking. The second type of lung cancer is adenocarcinoma, about 15% of the total, and a third
undifferentiated or anaplastic carcinoma, representing about 20% of all cases.
Epidermoid and adenocarcinoma are found primarily in smokers, and anaplastic
primarily in nonsmokers.

Lung cancer begins with the inhalation of carcinogenic material. The paralyzed
cilia cannot function to remove particles; thus tar is deposited on the respiratory
passageways and the tar and mucus buildup begins to attack the underlying epithelial
tissues. Cellular penetration of the constituents of smoke have been observed in the
laboratory.

This entire process takes time, usually 20 to 30 years. Early symptoms may be
a change in a chronic cough that the smoker may have had for years, fever, chills, an
increase in sputum production, and hemoptysis, or a wheeze. A worsening of these
symptoms indicates that the bronchiole obstruction has increased and there is a loss
of lung volume. Advanced-stage symptoms include weight loss, anorexia, nausea,
vomiting, and a generalized weakness. The longer the duration of symptoms, the
more likely the lesion is nonresectable; survival time for these cases varies from 5 to
14 months after diagnosis. Thirty to fifty percent prove to be treatable; of those
treated, about 20% survive for five years. In other words, if bronchogenic carcinoma
is diagnosed in 10 people, six will die within 14 months, and two within two to four
years, while the last two usually die during the fifth year.

Emphysema

Another lung ailment not well known at the turn of the century, but rapidly making
its presence felt as a smoking-related disease, is emphysema.

Emphysema is characterized by the rupture of alveolar (air sac) walls; this reduces the surface area in which gas exchange can take place (see Fig. 7.1 on page
121). Large pockets separated by scar tissue are formed, elasticity of the air sacs is
lost, and the emphysema victim finds it very difficult to release the air he or she has
taken into the lungs.

This is the emphysematic process in more detail: In a healthy individual, when
air is taken into the lungs, the bronchial passageways expand. Gas exchange (CO_2
from the tissues is exchanged for oxygen) then takes place in lung capillaries that
perfuse the millions of tiny air sacs throughout the lungs. Then the stale gases are
exhaled by virtue of pressure exerted on the lungs by the rib cage and diaphragm
and also by virtue of the elastic rebound of the air sacs and air passageways that
were stretched upon inhalation. This process is normally a simple, automatic one;

but in individuals who have an accumulation of cigarette tars (or other particula
matter such as coal dust) in their bronchial tubes, air is allowed in by the norm
expansion of the passageways and then is trapped because of the artificial blocki
agent—the tar that has accumulated over a period of time. Pressure builds up
the blocked-off structures, and tissues rupture, making large areas out of many sm;
ones. Scar tissue then develops, decreasing the elasticity of that area, so that
becomes even more difficult for the individual to exhale. It is not uncommon th
an emphysema patient cannot blow out a match held only an inch or two in front
his or her mouth. Emphysema victims become barrel-chested as a result of labore
exhalation, but gradually their increasing inability to exchange gases makes tl
remainder of their lives an agonizing effort.

In 1970 Hammond et al. [12] ended any remaining doubts concerning tl
relationship between smoking and emphysema. Beagles were taught to smoke cig
rettes and were exposed to various levels of tar and nicotine as they smoked eve
morning and afternoon for 875 days. The results clearly showed that fibrosis of tl
lung increased with exposure to higher tar and nicotine levels, as did the incidenc
and severity of emphysema. No emphysema was detected in the nonsmoking dog
Another classic study was conducted by Auerbach et al. [3], but this was an invest
gation of human lung sections from autopsies. They found that 90% of nonsmoke
had no emphysema, 47% of pipe and cigar smokers had no emphysema, 13%
who smoked less than one pack per day had no emphysema, and 0.3% who smoke
more than one pack per day had no emphysema.

Chronic bronchitis

Chronic bronchitis frequently precedes or accompanies emphysema. It is characte
ized by excessive mucus production in the bronchi of the lungs. The inflammatio
and hypersecretion of bronchi cells results in increased sputum and eventually
cough develops to remove the material that would normally be removed by ciliar
action. Although chronic bronchitis has been found in persons exposed to extrem
air pollution, coal dust, etc., the incidence in smokers is 20 times that in nonsmoke
and is greater in smokers who leave their cigarettes dangling from the lips betwee
puffs.

Smoking and pregnancy

From the preceding discussions on the relationship between smoking and physiolog
cal functions, it should be obvious that a developing fetus would also be affected.]
has been estimated that approximately one-third of the women in the United State
of childbearing age are smokers. Although not definitely known, it is estimated tha
only five to ten percent of these women quit smoking during pregnancy. Listed belo
are some of the most important findings related to smoking and pregnancy. Most ar
related to the effects of nicotine, but the polycyclic hydrocarbons (especially benzc
pyrene) have been found to reach the fetus [8, 9, 21, 22].

1. Cigarette smoking during pregnancy causes a reduction in infant birth weight.
2. Cigarette smoking is related to significantly higher fetal and neonatal mortality.
3. Cigarette smoking is associated with an increase in spontaneous abortions.
4. Preliminary study suggests that nicotine passes into the milk of lactating women; however, acute effects on the nursing infant have not yet been established.

Smoking and peptic ulcer

Statistical relationships have been established between smoking and the incidence of peptic ulcers. It has also been shown that smokers have a higher mortality rate from peptic ulcers than do nonsmokers. Nicotine has been found to inhibit pancreatic bicarbonate secretion, and it is believed that this mechanism is responsible for the potentiation of acute duodenal ulcer formation [17].

Pipe and cigar smoking

Mortality statistics show only a slight increase in health risk in pipe and cigar smokers when compared to nonsmokers. While this may give a sense of security to the pipe or cigar smoker, the feeling may be a bit premature. The ailments that seem to affect pipe and cigar smokers (cancer of the lip, oral cancer, cancer of the larynx, cancer of the esophagus, etc.) are easier to detect than cancer of the lung, treatment begins sooner, and thus, they cause relatively fewer deaths than does lung cancer.

Only small differences exist in the tobacco of cigarettes, cigars, and pipes. The primary difference lies in how the tobacco is used—mainly in the inhalation. Nicotine is absorbed into the bloodstream from the lungs, but it can also be absorbed from the lining of the oral cavity (but in significantly smaller amounts). Tars which cannot be washed from the bronchial lining can be largely eliminated from the oral cavity. However, tars will mix with saliva and be swallowed, giving rise to the increased incidence of stomach and urinary bladder cancer found in smokers.

Contrary to common belief, cigarette smokers have a higher incidence of oral cancer than do pipe or cigar smokers. Cigarette smokers who smoke pipes and cigars are more apt to inhale the smoke of the latter and do so more often than those individuals who smoke a pipe and/or cigars exclusively.

SUMMARY

Although 10 million Americans have quit smoking in the last five years, approximately 40% of adult Americans continue to smoke. Teenagers in increasing numbers begin smoking each year. Smoking is both a sociological and psychological phenomenon. It is a learned behavior, but satisfaction of psychological need and oral gratification create a positive reinforcement to continue. Reports have established beyond a doubt that smoking is harmful to the health of smokers and suggest that it is harmful to the persons around the smoker. Smoking-related diseases are the

most preventable known to our society, but knowledge of successful cessatic
methods still provides little competition against the seemingly strong motivation t
smoke.

REFERENCES

1. Althoff, S. A., and E. J. Nussel, "Social Class Trends in the Practice and Attitude
   of College Students Regarding Sex, Smoking, Drinking, and the Use of Drugs
   Journal of School Health, 8:445–447, 1971.

2. Astrup, P., "Tobacco Smoking and Coronary Disease," *Acta Cardiologica,* Supp
   20:105–117, 1974.

3. Auerbach, O., *et al.,* "Relation of Smoking and Age to Emphysema. Whole-Lun
   Section Study," *New England Journal of Medicine,* 286(16):653–657, 1972.

4. Best, J. A., "Tailoring Smoking Withdrawal Procedures to Personality and Motiva
   tional Differences," *Public Health,* 88(1):1–8, 1973.

5. Briney, K. L., *Cardiovascular Disease.* Belmont, Calif.: Wadsworth, 1970.

6. Castleden, C. M., *et al.,* "Variations in Carboxyhemoglobin Levels in Smokers,
   British Medical Journal, 4(5947):736–738, 1974.

7. Cellina, G. U., *et al.,* "Direct Arterial Pressure, Heart Rate, and Electrocardiogram
   During Cigarette Smoking in Unrestricted Patients," *American Heart Journal,* 89(1)
   18–25, 1975.

8. Colley, J. R. T., "Respiratory Symptoms in Children and Parental Smoking and
   Phlegm Production," *British Medical Journal,* 9:201–204, 1974.

9. Colley, J. R. T., *et al.,* "Influence of Passive Smoking and Parental Phlegm on Pneu
   monia and Bronchitis in Early Childhood," *British Medical Journal,* 2:1031–1034
   1974.

10. Diehl, H. S., *Tobacco and Your Health: the Smoking Controversy.* New York
    McGraw-Hill, 1974.

11. Goodman, L., and A. Gilman, "Tobacco (Nicotine)," in *Resource Book for Drug
    Abuse Education.* Chevy Chase, Md.: National Institute of Mental Health, 1969.

12. Hammond, E. C., *et al.,* "Effects of Cigarette Smoking on Dogs," *Archives of En
    vironmental Health,* 21:740–753, 1970.

13. Hasenfus, J. L., "Cigarettes and Health Education Among Young People," *Journa
    of School Health,* 41(7):372–376, 1971.

14. Hinds, W. C., *et al.,* "Concentrations of Nicotine and Tobacco Smoke in Public
    Places," *New England Journal of Medicine,* 292(16):844–845, 1975.

15. Iverson, N. T., "Smoke and Heat," *New England Journal of Medicine,* 293(1):47
    1975.

16. Jacobs, M. A., "Interaction of Personality and Treatment Conditions Associated
    with Success in a Smoking Control Program," *Psychosomatic Medicine,* 33(6):
    545–556, 1971.

17. Jedrychowski, W., *et al.,* "Association Between the Occurrence of Peptic Ulcers and
    Tobacco Smoking," *Public Health,* 88(4):195–200, 1974.

8. Kahn, E. B., and C. N. Edwards, "Smoking and Youth," *Journal of School Health,* 40(10):561–562, 1940.

9. Kroll, H. W., "Bibliography on Behavioral Approaches to Modification of Smoking: January 1964 through December 1973," *Psychological Reports,* 35:435–440, 1974.

0. McRae, C. F., and D. M. Nelson, "Youth to Youth Communication of Smoking and Health," *Journal of School Health,* 41(8):445–447, 1971.

1. Meyer, M. B., *et al.,* "The Interrelationship of Maternal Smoking and Increased Perinatal Mortality with Other Risk Factors,"· *American Journal of Epidemiology,* 100(6):443–452, 1974.

2. Miller, H. C., *et al.,* "Maternal Smoking and Fetal Growth of Full Term Infants," *Pediatric Research,* 8(12):960–963, 1974.

3. Newman, I. M., "Adolescent Cigarette Smoking as Compensatory Behavior," *Journal of School Health,* 40(6):316–321, 1970.

4. Newman, I. M., "Ninth Grade Smokers—Two Years Later," *Journal of School Health,* 41(9):497–501, 1971.

5. Newman, I. M., "Status Configuration and Cigarette Smoking in a Junior High School," *Journal of School Health,* 41(1):28–32, 1971.

6. Pflaum, J., "Smoking Behavior," *Journal of Applied Behavioral Science,* 1(2):195–209, 1965.

7. Pierre, R. S., *et al.,* "Reducing Smoking Using Positive Self-Management," *Journal of School Health,* 45(1):709, 1975.

8. Russell, M. A., "Blood and Urinary Nicotine in Nonsmokers," *Lancet,* 1(7905):527, 1975.

9. Schmeltz, I., *et al.,* "The Influence of Tobacco Smoke on Indoor Atmospheres," *Preventive Medicine,* 4(1):66–82, 1975.

30. Spain, D. M., *et al.,* "Women Smokers and Sudden Death: the Relationship of Cigarette Smoking to Coronary Disease," *Journal of the American Medical Association,* 224(7):1005–1007, 1973.

31. Wilson, D. G., "Mental Effects of Secondhand Smoke," *New England Journal of Medicine,* 292(11):596, 1975.

SUGGESTED READING

Brody, A. R., *et al.,* "Cytoplasmic Inclusions in Pulmonary Macrophages in Cigarette Smokers," *Laboratory Investigation,* 32(2):125–132, 1975.

Eysenck, H. J., *Smoking, Health and Personality.* New York: Basic Books, 1965.

Hickey, R. J., *et al.,* "Cigarette Smoking as a Carcinogen?" *American Review of Respiratory Diseases,* 111(1):105–106, 1975.

Horn, Daniel, "Man, Cigarettes, and the Abuse of Gratification," *Archives of Environmental Health,* 20:88–92, 1970.

Lichenstein, E., "How to Quit Smoking," *Psychology Today,* 4:44–45, 1971.

Magnuson, W. G., and J. Carper, "Toward a Safer Cigarette," in W. G. Magnuson and

J. Carper, eds., *The Dark Side of the Market Place,* pp. 185–207. Englewood Cliffs, N.J. Prentice-Hall, 1968.

Martin, R. R., *et al.,* "Reversible Small Airway Obstruction Associated with Cigarett Smoking," *Chest,* 63:315, 1973.

Neeman, R. L., *et al.,* "Complexities of Smoking Education," *Journal of School Healtl* 45(1):17–23, 1975.

Newman, A. N., "How Teachers See Themselves in the Exemplar Role in Smoking ε Evidenced by their Attitudes and Practices," *Journal of School Health,* 41(5):275–27￥ 1971.

Oakes, T. W., *et al.,* "Health Service Utilization by Smokers and Nonsmokers," *Medicε Care,* 12(11):958–966, 1974.

Scheiderman, M. A., and D. L. Levin, "Trends in Lung Cancer Mortality Diagnosi￥ Treatment, Smoking and Urbanization," *Cancer,* 30(5):1320–1325, 1972.

Schievelbein, H., and R. Eberhardt, "Cardiovascular Actions of Nicotine and Smoking, *Journal of the National Cancer Institute,* 48(6):1785–1794, 1972.

Shryock, H., *Mind If I Smoke.* Mountain View, Calif.: Pacific Press Publication, 197(

United States Department of Health, Education, and Welfare, *Smoking and Healtl* Washington, D.C.: U.S. Government Printing Office, 1974.

Weir, J. M., and J. E. Dunn, Jr., "Smoking and Mortality: A Prospective Study," *Cance* 25:105–112, 1970.

Wynder, E. L., and K. Mabuchi, "Lung Cancer Among Cigar and Pipe Smokers," *Pre ventive Medicine,* 1(4):529–542, 1972.

8 BARBITURATES AND NONBARBITURATE SEDATIVES

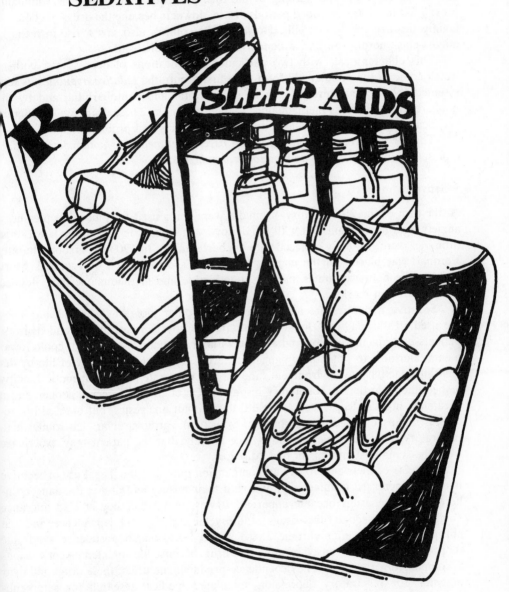

GENERAL INFORMATION

As the drug revolution swept through the country, marijuana and the psychedelic played both cause and effect roles. Then as the counterculture continued, it saw the "freak-fringe" people turning to the thrill of speed. And when the stimulant proved too harsh for extended periods of use, downers became the drugs of choice— mainly through the use of pills. However, the country also saw a rise in teenage middle-class heroin use and a concurrent rise in alcoholism.

This chapter deals with two particular classifications of depressants, both of which come in the popular pill form. The first group, the *sedative hypnotics,* is represented by the barbiturates such as secobarbital and pentobarbital, and by the nonbarbiturates such as methaqualone and glutethimide. These drugs are of different chemical formulations, but all produce similar effects and problems.

The second group, commonly called *psychotherapeutic* or *antianxiety drugs,* is represented by the *major and minor tranquilizers.*

Sedative hypnotics

At the turn of the 20th century, bromides were being used to combat sleeplessness, anxiety, and minor pain, but with the discovery of barbituric acid in the late 1800s bromides were gradually replaced with the barbiturates. In 1903 the first barbiturate Veronal, was placed on the market, and it was soon followed by Luminal. More recently the nonbarbiturates such as glutethimide and methaqualone have flooded the prescription market.

Sedative hypnotics are among the most popular tools of the physician. They are used (1) in daytime, low-dose sedative therapy to treat normal and neurotic patients by reducing tension and anxiety without inducing lethargy that could lower mental alertness to potentially dangerous levels or reduce the quality of life by decreasing reactivity to environment, and (2) in moderate-dose or hypnotic therapy at bedtime in order to counteract insomnia. Onset of sleep occurs sooner and a dreamless night's sleep ensues. These drugs are not analgesics, but often aid in reducing the psychological component involved in cardiovascular, gastrointestinal, respiratory, or other diseases and reduce anxiety that the patient may experience from the somatic symptoms of these diseases.

Because of their antianxiety and antitension qualities, the illegal use of sedative hypnotics increased dramatically, and with their misuse and abuse, the dangers inherent in these drugs became apparent. It was found that they created tolerance (and cross-tolerance to other drugs) and psychic and physical dependence, and that abrupt withdrawal after chronic abuse would bring on an abstinence syndrome more severe than that caused by any other drug, because life-threatening convulsions accompanied withdrawal. The dependence-producing nature of these drugs and their potential for respiratory depression stimulated medical research for safer substances. The drugs that emerged from this research were the tranquilizers, most of which unfortunately possess potential dangers identical to the sedative hypnotics— tolerance, dependence, and overdose.

The sedative hypnotics produce their depressant effect by inhibiting the arousal system of the central nervous system; that is, they depress the reticular formation by interfering with oxygen consumption and energy-producing mechanisms. The depression here reduces the nerve signals that reach the cortex, thus promoting sleep. A sedative dose makes one only slightly drowsy, but damps out enough incoming stimuli to reduce anxiety and tension.

The body eliminates sedative hypnotics via the kidneys at varying rates, and it is mainly this rate of elimination that determines the duration effects of any one drug. There is an exception here in that short- and ultrashort-acting barbiturates rapidly redistribute themselves in adipose tissue, thus lessening their levels and effects in the brain. The intermediate- and long-acting drugs are metabolized more slowly and may produce some residual sedation (hangover) because they have not been thoroughly metabolized.

An interesting paradox with these drugs is that abusive levels in chronic users or normal doses in susceptible patients, especially the elderly, can produce excitation before the customary depressant action sets in. Another interesting effect of barbiturates is that when taken in the presence of psychological stress or extreme pain, they may cause delirium and other side effects such as nausea, nervousness, rash, and diarrhea [16]. Another adverse effect of barbiturates, glutethimide, and other drugs of this classification is that they decrease the potency of certain anticoagulant drugs.

Tranquilizers

The tranquilizers are divided into antipsychotic and antianxiety substances, also commonly known as the major and minor tranquilizers, respectively. The difference between these two groups of tranquilizers is of significance, for the major tranquilizers (drugs such as Thorazine and Reserpine) hold no hazard of physical dependence and are not street drugs of misuse or abuse. Thorazine (generic name, chlorpromazine) is the drug of choice in most mental hospitals for alleviating the symptoms of psychosis and rendering patients more susceptible to therapy. The remainder of this chapter refers only to the minor tranquilizers which, like the sedative hypnotics, are common drugs of misuse and abuse. The rise in consumption of tranquilizers began in the 1960s with Miltown and Equanil (generic name, meprobamate) as the prototypes, and these were later replaced by Librium and Valium. In 1968 40 million prescriptions were written for these latter two drugs. Five years later the number was 80 million, about eight percent of all prescriptions written by physicians in the United States. (More prescriptions are written for tranquilizers than for any other psychoactive drug!) The implications here are that many Americans are trying to solve their problems through the use of psychotropic drugs, and that American physicians feel that tranquilizers are the most efficient manner in which to deal with their anxiety-ridden patients. The all-out prescribing of tranquilizers has its impact on the street drug scene in two ways—directly, by supplying legitimate drugs (via theft) to the black market system, and indirectly, through parental example of attitudes toward drugs. Use of illicit drugs by teenagers has been shown to parallel their parents' use of tranquilizers, with children being especially influenced by their mothers' use of these drugs.

The action of tranquilizers on the central nervous system is quite dissimilar to that of the sedative hypnotics. Rather than suppress activity of the reticular activating system, the tranquilizers act on the limbic system, which is involved in emotional response. Experimental research has shown a "taming" action of tranquilizers on hostile and vicious animals and subsequent anxiety reduction in humans. These drugs are depressants and at higher than normal dosage levels can cause sedation or death from overdose, and will potentiate other depressant drugs.

The drugs of concern in this chapter are characterized by those listed in Table 8.1. Those that appear have been selected for description because of their incidence of high abuse. There are, of course, countless other barbiturates, nonbarbiturates, and tranquilizers on the market. If taken in excessive doses over a long enough period of time, all of the drugs that are listed will create tolerance and physical and psychological dependence.

DANGERS OF MISUSE

From currently available information we find that (a) as seen in Fig. 8.1, the drugs in question are dangerous drugs, (b) the supply exceeds the demand [30], and (c) these drugs do not solve problems of anxiety—they merely treat the symptoms. In view of these facts, we wonder why pharmaceutical companies continue to manufacture them and doctors continue to prescribe them. Meares [20] has suggested three answers to the latter question, the first being that a barbiturate prescription occasionally relieves the anxiety of physicians who feel that unless they prescribe something for their patients, they are not doing their duty. Second, even though the physician knows that insomnia or anxiety is a symptom of a deeper inner conflict, he or she may not have sufficient time to help resolve the patient's real problem. Hence, a prescription is made out to treat the symptom. Third, either the physician may be unwilling to use new drugs or is not up to date on current medicine.

In prescribing sedative hypnotics or tranquilizers to a patient who is in an anxious state of mind, the physician is placing a dangerous drug in the hands of a person who, in his or her mental state, may be dependence- or suicide-prone.

Alteration of sleep patterns

A real drawback of prescribing the sedative hypnotics for relief of insomnia is that many of these drugs reduce REM (rapid eye movement) sleep time. It appears that REM sleep is necessary, for if individuals are deprived of this period of sleep in which dreams occur, they grow irritable, anxious, and even neurotic. In a normal night's sleep, five or six periods of orthodox sleep occur broken up by short periods of REM sleep, with the first period occurring about an hour to an hour and a half after onset of sleep and lasting varying lengths of time. Normally, REM sleep makes up 20% to 25% of one's total sleep time [3, 14].

TABLE 8.1
Barbiturates, nonbarbiturates, and minor tranquilizers of high abuse—their description, normal dosage, and use [5].

Drug	Description	Normal dose and use
Barbiturates of high abuse		
Amobarbital sodium (Amytal, Lilly*)	65 or 200 mg blue capsule	30–50 mg for sedation 100–200 mg for hypnosis
Sodium pentobarbital (Nembutal, Abbott*)	30 or 100 mg yellow capsule	30–50 mg for sedation 100 mg for hypnosis
Secobarbital (Seconal, Lilly*)	30, 50, or 100 mg red capsule	100 mg for insomnia
(Tuinal, Lilly*)	50, 100, or 200 mg capsule, blue body with red-orange cap	50–200 mg for insomnia
Nonbarbiturates		
Glutethimide (Doriden, Ciba*)	125, 250, or 500 mg white tablet, "Ciba" inscribed	125–250 mg for sedation 500 mg for hypnosis
Methyprylon (Noludar, Roche*)	300 mg capsule, pink cap and white bottom	300 mg for insomnia
Ethchlorynol (Placidyl, Abbott*)	100, 200 mg red tablet 500 mg red capsule 750 mg green capsule	100–200 mg for sedation 500 mg for hypnosis
Methaqualone (Quaalude, Rorer*)	150, 300 mg white tablet	75 mg for sedation 150–300 mg for insomnia
Tranquilizers		
Meprobamate (Miltown, Wallace*)	200, 400 mg white tablet	400–800 mg for anxiety and tension
(Equanil, Wyeth*)	200 mg white pentagonal tablet 400 mg white round tablet	400 mg for simple anxiety and tension
Chlordiazepoxide (Librium, Roche*)	5 mg capsule green top, yellow 10 mg capsule green top, black 25 mg capsule green top, white	5–10 mg for mild to moderate anxiety and tension 20–25 mg for severe anxiety and tension
Diazepam (Valium, Roche*)	2 mg white tablet 5 mg yellow tablet 10 mg baby blue tablet	2–5 mg for moderate psychoneurotic reactions 5–10 mg for severe reactions

* Brand name and pharmaceutical company.

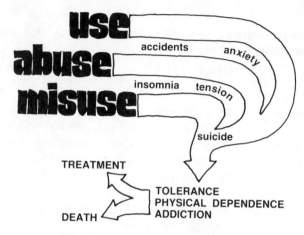

Fig. 8.1   Dangers of sedative use.

Unfortunately, the use of barbiturates as a sleeping aid creates an initial reduction of REM sleep, which occurs during the first week of nighttime hypnosis. Subsequent nightly use of barbiturates for as little as two weeks [23] brings about some tolerance; it takes longer to fall asleep and total sleep time is shorter, but REM sleep time rises to normal levels again. Even though one regains a normal level of REM sleep, a serious situation has arisen with the REM sleep that was lost initially. It has been found that there is a large increase in REM sleep after one discontinues using sleeping pills [3, 4, 14, 20, 26]. When this increase occurs, patients experience nightmares, restlessness, and nighttime awakenings. They feel they do not get a full night's sleep and become anxious about their poor sleeping behavior. This situation is very likely to induce patients to return to barbiturates to "cure" the problem. Study has shown that it takes a month or more to repay this REM sleep debt [4, 23]; but if the patient can withstand the transition period, he can escape the barbiturate-induced sleep routine.

A number of drug researchers have suggested the use of Nitrazepam as a substitute drug for barbiturates in cases of insomnia and other neurotic symptoms, because this drug appears to have fewer adverse effects [13, 19, 20, 22].

Suicide and accidental death

Other dangers in the use of sedative hypnotics and, to some extent, tranquilizers as well are suicide and accidental death. In the United States barbiturates are the leading prescription drug used for suicide; in the United Kingdom barbiturates have been recently found to be the mode of suicide in two-thirds of all suicides; in Australia 83% of a series of impulsive suicides have involved barbiturates as the means of death [21].

In many cases it is difficult to determine whether death was accidental or planned, because the effects of drug poisoning occur gradually. Termination of life is not instantaneous. Thus insomniacs who take one or two sleeping pills and find that these do not work immediately may take more. If the second dose added to the first exceeds the lethal dose for the individual, death will occur. Another way in which suicide or accidental death occurs is through self-administration of sedative hypnotics or tranquilizers after ingesting a large amount of alcohol [7]. The lethal dose of these depressants is markedly reduced in such a case because alcohol has already depressed vital cell action. Similar effects occur with any multiple drug use which is a combination of depressant drugs; barbiturates and opiates, methaqualone and alcohol, or alcohol and methadone, for example.

Another hazard is that of operating dangerous machinery, especially an automobile, while under the influence of sedative drugs. Barbiturates and similar drugs cause a type of intoxication that is much like alcohol intoxication; the individual initially experiences a relaxed feeling, and release of social inhibitions occurs, just as in the first stages of alcohol intoxication. Further use of the drug brings on sluggishness, lack of motor coordination, slurred speech, and eventually sleep. However, large doses of these drugs in the stomach do not affect the vomiting mechanism as large amounts of alcohol do (rescuing the drunk from death); thus large doses of barbiturates, for example, are more dangerous than alcohol.

All the dangers described here (loss of REM sleep, death by accident or suicide, potentiation of other drugs) stem from misuse of barbiturates or barbituratelike drugs. There is the additional danger that misuse will lead to an ever-increasing *abuse* of these drugs; that is, instead of misusing legal prescriptions, individuals may buy these drugs illegally purely for psychological gratification. There are three factors that lend support to the idea that misuse is the forerunner of abuse. First, without these drugs of increasingly dubious medical value, there would be no overflow of the drug itself into channels of abuse. In the United States in one year, six billion 60-mg capsules of barbiturates alone are manufactured [21], and methaqualone production went from 8 million doses in 1968 to 105 million in 1972. The AMA Committee on Alcoholism and Addiction suggests that current production of all sedatives exceeds medical needs by a considerable margin. Granted, a drug alone does not create drug abuse; but a second point is that these drugs are prescribed mainly to individuals who are in a weakened psychological condition. Misuse during this low period may lead to future abuse. Third, the widespread medical use of these drugs gives them an air of universal acceptance, such as alcohol is given, thus aiding the development of our whole drug culture.

Taking all three factors (the drug, the individual, and the culture) into consideration, one might conclude that these drugs should not be so freely prescribed. It is an interesting sidelight and comment on our culture that the majority of current barbiturate and tranquilizer research is being done in Australia, the United Kingdom, and various other foreign countries. Very little appears in the American medical journals. Is this a reflection of our disinterest, a reflection on vested interests, an indication that researching the more spectacular and currently controversial drugs is more rewarding, or are there other reasons for this lack of research in the United States?

DANGERS OF ABUSE

Abuse of the sedatives is a more intense problem than misuse of these drugs because of the more serious physical, psychological, and social dangers involved. Goodman and Gilman [8] say that persons with a tendency to become addicted to barbiturates have some basic personality disorder or psychoneurosis. They also feel that this type of addiction presents a greater public health and mental problem than heroin addiction because it produces more severe emotional, mental, and neurological problems and withdrawal is more dangerous.

The American Medical Association has provided a breakdown or categorization of the different types of individuals who abuse sedative drugs. It will be easy to recognize that these individuals differ from the common misuser described earlier in the chapter, the difference being mainly the *intensity* of motive and dosage. The categories are as follows:

1. Those who seek sedative effects to deal with emotional stress. This sedation may be carried to extremes when the person seeks almost total oblivion and stupor, moving about only to answer nature's call or to take more drugs.

2. Another group seeks the paradoxical excitation that has been seen to occur, especially after one can tolerate large doses of the drug. Now instead of depression, the person feels exhilaration—much like the initial effect of amphetamines—and uses the drug for typical stimulatory reasons.

3. Many sedative users take the drug to counteract the effects of abusive use of stimulants and LSD. This kind of use may set up a cycle of ups and downs that eventually leads to addiction.

4. There is a group that uses sedatives in combination with other depressant drugs, mainly alcohol and heroin. Alcohol plus the sedative gives a more instant "high" but is especially dangerous because of the double depressant action. Heroin users often resort to barbiturates if their heroin supply is cut off [1].

The four categories given above probably overlap very little and give a fairly good picture of the various types of abusers. The solution for all of these individuals has to be realignment of values based on factual knowledge.

Tolerance and physical dependence

Two of the most dangerous aspects of barbiturate abuse are those of physical and psychological dependence. If an individual takes barbiturates as prescribed, dependence is not likely to occur (however, tolerance to even small doses may develop). For various reasons, though, people may increase their dose of barbiturates and build their tolerance to incredible levels. When this occurs and the barbiturate or tranquilizer is taken regularly, true addiction will develop (see Fig. 8.2).

It is commonly recognized that two factors, *tolerance* and *physical dependence* (and a third, psychological dependence), are necessary for true addiction to occur, and although they have been intensely studied for over half a century, their precise

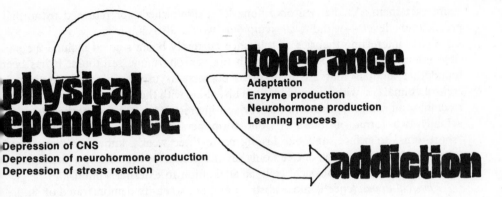

Fig. 8.2 The pattern of addiction.

mechanisms of action are not understood. Nonetheless, their existence is an inescapable fact for all too many abusers of depressant drugs.

Even though the exact mechanisms are not known, the literature on this subject does not suffer from a lack of hypothesized causes of tolerance and dependence. While it is not our purpose here to discuss all of these theories, some will be outlined briefly in an attempt to explain the all-important cellular control over these phenomena.

Tolerance and physical dependence are presented together because, though not necessarily interdependent, they are definitely interrelated. *Tolerance* has been characterized as *diminished cellular response to repeated exposure to a drug*. This, of course, means that it takes more of the drug to produce the same effects. Tolerance is basically adaptation. In a general sense, the ability of the human organism to adapt is one of its most significant survival mechanisms [24], but in the present context tolerance must be considered a "disease" of adaptation.

Since the lethal dose of barbiturates does not increase as tolerance to these drugs increases, some have considered the ability to function in the face of ever-increasing depression of the central nervous system a learning process [15]. Although learning or adaptation on a cognitive level is undoubtedly part of the tolerance phenomenon, researchers have found evidence of physical changes as well. One such change is in the activity of the liver's drug-metabolizing enzymes. As the intake of barbiturates increases, so does the activity of the liver enzymes that break down the drug. As time goes on, increasing quantities of the drug must be ingested in order to have the same amount of the drug circulating in the system [28, 29].

Another enzymatic theory was proposed by Shuster [25], who indicated that initial depression of neurohormone-producing systems (that is, systems for production of norepinephrine, serotonin, etc.) caused the body to overproduce these hormones so that the natural, normal (pre-drug) levels could be maintained. Therefore, increased drug dosage would be necessary to overcome the increased levels of neurohormones. Withdrawal symptoms, then, are due to the high level of neurohormones that would be present when the depressant drug was no longer there to counteract them. As the neurohormone level diminished—or returned to normal, preaddiction levels—withdrawal symptoms would also diminish.

Other interesting theories of tolerance currently being studied include the possible interaction of the depressants with the neurohormone serotonin. It has been found that animals that are tolerant to depressants use more serotonin than do control animals or withdrawn animals. This, along with the hypothesis that tolerance resembles an immune reaction, has revived interest in an old theory that there are actually two forms of tolerance: one form persisting up to eight hours, called "short-term" tolerance, and one lasting up to three weeks, known as "long-term" tolerance [2]. In summary, one can only say that tolerance is basically a phenomenon of biochemical and biophysical cellular adaptation to external stimuli.

Physical dependence is more abstract and not so easily demonstrated or studied as tolerance. A unique biological phenomenon characterized by a *metabolic demand for a particular substance,* it has been described as a state of pseudohomeostasis—a hyperexcitability that develops in the cells of the central nervous system after prolonged use of depressants such as heroin, alcohol, or barbituratelike substances. However, this phenomenon can be seen only when the depressant is withheld, and symptoms known as the *abstinence* or *withdrawal syndrome* emerge [24].

Theories presented to explain physical dependence generally center on (a) the production, release, and/or destruction of neurohormones (such as norepinephrine), (b) neuronal sensitivity, and (c) depression of endocrine function [18].

Because of similarities in the abstinence syndrome caused by such chemically dissimilar agents as alcohol, barbiturates, meprobamate, paraldehyde, chlordiazepoxide, and others—and because these substances have the capacity to stave off signs of withdrawal in users of other depressants, including heroin, due to cross-tolerance—one mechanism for physical dependence seems to be depression of nervous activity in similar central nervous system pathways [6]. This may be initial depression at the synapse followed by a gradual limiting of the production of neurohormones. As one pathway becomes depressed, other parallel, or redundant, pathways may enlarge their function and continue body processes on a somewhat depressed level [11, 17]. The body's amazing homeostasis or equilibrium-maintaining mechanisms (centered primarily in the hypothalamus) allow for continued functioning without triggering stress reactions. This results in a sort of disease of adaptation (theories of tolerance here interact with the theory of physical dependence). This adaptation affects the endocrine glands, which are depressed and therefore do not produce the stress reactions that usually accompany altered homeostatic conditions.

Upon withdrawal of the depressant there is extreme hyperexcitability, due in part to release of depressed stress reactions and in part to restoration of depressed neural pathways. In essence, the body is now able to realize to what extent its homeostasis or equilibrium has been altered, and violent stress reactions (the classic withdrawal symptoms) are now felt. As outlined by Wulff [31], this first appears as a sense of apprehension and general weakness, which soon develops into muscle fasciculations, tremors of the hands, hyperactive reflexes, insomnia, abdominal cramps, nausea, and vomiting. There is an extreme dehydration and rapid loss of eight accompanied by increases in heart rate, blood pressure, and respiratory rate. Disorientation in time and space, hallucinations, and death are not uncommon.

It has been widely observed that development of physical dependence on barbiturates is a relatively slow process requiring weeks or months before withdrawal symptoms are manifested. Doses of 200 mg to 400 mg of pentobarbital or secobarbital can be taken daily for a year with little or no physical dependence resulting. It would take daily doses between 900 and 2000 mg for one month to produce withdrawal symptoms as described above [6]. However, it has been demonstrated more recently that large doses of short-acting pentobarbital can produce some mild withdrawal symptoms after only 26 hours of intoxication, with symptoms increasing in severity as the length of intoxication increases [11]. Taking 300 mg to 600 mg of Librium per day for five months will produce physical dependence with serious withdrawal; Doriden, secobarbital, and pentobarbital at around one gram per day for a month or more, Miltown at 1.5–2.5 grams per day for a prolonged period, or methaqualone at two to three grams per day for a month will produce a similar dependence.

Treatment

The treatment for withdrawal from sedative drugs is one of intensive care and should be carried out in a hospital, where every medical advantage may be gained over the possibly fatal withdrawal symptoms. Many addicts who enter a hospital for treatment are also addicted to heroin. In such cases, withdrawal from the barbituatelike drug is the major focus, with heroin treatment following [27].

Addicts seek treatment when they can no longer cope with the sedative-induced depression, when they are arrested, when they can no longer afford their drug habits, or for a number of other reasons. Upon commencing treatment, if withdrawal has begun, the individual will appear weak, anxious, nauseous, and/or tremulous. These symptoms signal the danger of convulsion and/or psychosis. If the patient does not yet show these symptoms, a careful vigil is kept so that they can be treated immediately upon their onset.

In the first eight hours after abrupt withdrawal, signs of intoxication decline and the patient's condition actually appears to improve. However, after eight hours the symptoms described above occur, perhaps accompanied by signs such as muscle twitches, impaired cardiovascular responses, headache, and vomiting. These signs and symptoms increase in intensity for the next eight hours (until about 16 hours after withdrawal from the drug) and become quite severe after 24 hours. Untreated, these conditions will likely develop into *grand mal*-type seizures between the thirtieth and forty-eighth hours. These convulsive seizures have been seen as early as the sixteenth hour and as late as the eighth day after abrupt withdrawal [1].

During and following these two days there may be recurrences of insomnia culminating in delirium (much like the delirium tremens), hallucinations, disorientation, and marked tremors. The delirium typically lasts about five days, ending with a long, deep sleep. The whole withdrawal process is self-limiting, even if untreated. However, death is a real danger in uncontrolled, untreated withdrawal [9].

Treatment usually consists of administering an initial short-acting barbiturate (usually pentobarbital) to allay the first symptoms of withdrawal and then tapering off either with the same drug [1] or with continually decreased doses of a long-acting drug [27]. Because there is a cross-tolerance with many of these drugs, theoretically any of them could be administered during the withdrawal process. The treatment that involves tapering doses of a short-acting barbiturate consists of administering 200–400 mg of sodium pentobarbital when withdrawal symptoms initially appear. Subsequent treatment calls for a graduated four-times-daily administration of the same barbiturate, at a dosage just strong enough to maintain a mild degree of intoxication (usually 200–300 mg of sodium pentobarbital is sufficient). After one or two days of observation, the dose level can again be reduced (not to less than 100 mg daily, however).

This treatment, described by the AMA Committee on Alcoholism and Addiction [1], is combined with supportive measures such as vitamin administration, restoration of electrolyte balance, and proper hydration. A close vigil is still kept on the patient because apprehension, mental confusion, and mental incompetence will likely occur during treatment.

Smith et al. [27] describe a different plan of sedative-drug withdrawal treatment which has been found successful at the San Francisco General Hospital. Supportive treatment is given as just described, but instead of short-acting barbiturates administered four times a day, a number of sedative doses equivalent to the number of hypnotic doses the addict was taking daily is given at six-hour intervals. Instead of the short-acting drug, the long-acting phenobarbital is used. After two days of this treatment, the dose is gradually diminished in specific decrements over an eight-day period. Smith and his colleagues point out that this technique can be used for withdrawal from meprobamate (Miltown) or glutethimide (Doriden), since withdrawal symptoms of these drugs follow the same pattern and entail the same dangers [12]. This is likewise true for methaqualone and the minor tranquilizers.

Detoxification is often the only aspect of treatment for barbiturate withdrawal considered. This, however, is only the beginning. After medical treatment assures the patient that he or she is no longer physically addicted to the drug, help must be given to the patient to keep his or her psychological state from causing a relapse into drug use. This process of psychological and social rehabilitation is similar to that used for the heroin addict, described in Chapter 9.

First-aid treatment

In addition to hospital treatment during withdrawal, first-aid measures are often necessary, especially in cases of drug overdose. Since barbiturates, nonbarbiturate sedatives, and the tranquilizers are often abused, because the various kinds may be taken at the same time, and because they may be taken with alcohol, overdoses are not uncommon.

In a victim of barbiturate overdose, for example, coma, flaccidity of the muscles, and respiratory depression would likely be apparent. The treatment to follow would be to (a) open the airway and clear out the oral cavity, (b) give mouth-to-mouth esuscitation if breathing has stopped, and (c) check the pulse. If there is no pulse, perform cardioresuscitative procedures [10].

If withdrawal symptoms are apparent (convulsions or preconvulsion symptoms), the same emergency measures should be followed with the possible addition of (d) intravenous administration of a drug such as diazepam at a very slow rate. This last step is not to be performed by nonmedical or nonparamedical personnel.

REFERENCES

1. AMA Committee on Alcoholism and Addiction, "Dependence on Barbiturates and Other Sedative Drugs," *Journal of the American Medical Association,* 193:673–677, 1965.

2. Cochin, J., "Possible Mechanisms in Development of Tolerance," *Federation Proceedings, Federation of American Societies for Experimental Biology,* 29:19–27, 1970.

3. Davison, K., *et al.,* "A Comparison of Sleep Patterns in Natural and Mandrax- and Tuinal-Induced Sleep," *Canadian Medical Journal,* 102:506–508, 1970.

4. Evans, J. I., *et al.,* "Sleep and Barbiturates: Some Experiments and Observations," *British Medical Journal,* 4:291–293, 1968.

5. Folsom, J. P. (Gen. Mgr.), *Physicians' Desk Reference to Pharmaceutical Specialties and Biologicals.* Oradell, N.J.: Medical Economics, Inc., 1970.

6. Fraser, H. F., *et al.,* "Degree of Physical Dependence Induced by Secobarbital or Pentobarbital," *Journal of the American Medical Association,* 166:126, 1958.

7. Fraser, H. F., *et al.,* "Partial Equivalence of Chronic Alcohol and Barbiturate Intoxications," *Quarterly Journal of Studies on Alcohol,* 18:541, 1957.

8. Goodman, L. S., and A. Gilman, *The Pharmacological Basis of Therapeutics,* 3rd ed. New York: Macmillan, 1965.

9. Hadden, J., "Acute Barbiturate Intoxication," *Journal of the American Medical Association,* 209:893–899, 1969.

10. Haight-Ashbury Free Medical Clinic, "The Treatment of Acute Drug Overdose," Indianapolis: Eli Lilly.

11. Jaffe, J. H., and S. K. Sharpless, "The Rapid Development of Physical Dependence on Barbiturates," *Journal of Pharmacology and Experimental Therapeutics,* 150:140–145, 1965.

12. Johnson, F. A., and H. C. Van Buren, "Abstinence Syndrome Following Glutethimide Intoxication," *Journal of the American Medical Association,* 180:1024–1027, 1962.

13. Johnson, J., and A. D. Clift, "Dependence on Hypnotic Drugs in General Practice," *British Medical Journal,* 4:613–617, 1968.

14. Kales, A., ed., *Sleep: Physiology and Pathology. A Symposium.* Philadelphia: Lippincott, 1969.

15. Kayan, S., *et al.,* "Experience as a Factor in the Development of Tolerance," *European Journal of Pharmacology,* 6:333–339, 1969.

16. Lingeman, R. R., *Drugs from A to Z: a Dictionary*. New York: McGraw-Hill, 197.

17. Martin, W. R., "Pharmacological Redundancy as an Adaptive Mechanism in th Central Nervous System," *Federation Proceedings, Federation of American Societie for Experimental Biology*, 29:13–18, 1970.

18. McBride, A., and M. J. Turnbull, "The Brain Acetylcholine System in Barbitone Dependent and Withdrawn Rats," *British Journal of Pharmacology*, 39:210p-211p 1970.

19. McQueen, E. G., "Dangers of Barbiturates," *British Medical Journal*, 2:295, 197C

20. Meares, R., "The Place of Barbiturates in Psychiatric Treatment," *Medical Journa of Australia*, 1:1207–1209, 1970.

21. Milner, G., "Interaction between Barbiturates, Alcohol, and some Psychotropi Drugs," *Medical Journal of Australia*, 1:1204–1206, 1970.

22. Mitchell, N., and T. Christopher, "The Effects of Prescribing Minimal Barbiturate in an Acute Psychiatric Ward," *British Journal of Psychiatry*, 112:733–735, 1966

23. Oswald, I., and R. G. Priest, "Five Weeks to Escape the Sleeping Pill Habit," *Britis Medical Journal*, 2:1093, 1965.

24. Seevers, M. H., and G. A. Deneau, "Physiological Aspects of Tolerance and Physica Dependence," in W. S. Root and F. G. Hofmann, eds., *Physiological Pharmacology* New York: Academic Press, 1963.

25. Shuster, L., "Repression and De-repression of Enzyme Synthesis as a Possible Ex planation of Some Aspects of Drug Action," *Nature*, 189:314–315, 1961.

26. "Sleep Now, Pay Later" (Editorial), *Journal of the American Medical Association* 208:1485, 1969.

27. Smith, D. E., *et al.*, "New Developments in Barbiturate Abuse," in D. E. Smith, ed. *Drug Abuse Papers*. Berkeley: University of California Press, 1969.

28. Stevenson, J. H., and M. J. Turnbull, "Hepatic Drug-Metabolism Enzyme Activity and Duration of Hexobarbitone Anaesthesia," *Biochemical Pharmacology*, 17:2297– 2305, 1968.

29. Stevenson, J. H., and M. J. Turnbull, "Sensitivity of the Brain to Barbiturates," *British Journal of Pharmacology*, 39:325–333, 1970.

30. United States Senate Hearings, *Methaqualone (Quaalude, Sopor) Traffic, Abuse, and Regulation*. Washington, D.C.: U.S. Government Printing Office, 1973.

31. Wulff, M. H., "The Barbiturate Withdrawal Syndrome: a Clinical and Electro- encephalographic Study," *Electroencephalography and Clinical Neurophysiology*, Supp. 14, 1959.

SUGGESTED READING

Anumonye, A., "Personality Factors and Barbiturate Dependence," *British Journal of Addiction*, 64:365–370, 1970.

Benson, W. M., and B. C. Schiele, *Tranquilizing and Anti-depressive Drugs*. Springfield, Ill.: Charles C. Thomas, 1962.

Brooke, E. M., and M. M. Glatt, "More and More Barbiturates," *Medical Science Law,* 4:277–282, 1964.

Brophy, J. J., "Suicide Attempts with Psychotherapeutic Drugs," *Archives of General Psychiatry,* 17:642, 1967.

Caldwell, J., *et al.,* "The Biochemical Pharmacology of Abused Drugs II. Alcohol and Barbiturates," *Clinical Pharmacology and Therapeutics,* 16(5):737–749, 1974.

Chambers, C. D., "Barbiturate-Sedative Abuse: a Study of Prevalence among Narcotic Abusers," *International Journal of the Addictions,* 4:45–58, 1969.

Cumberlidge, M. C., "Abuse of Barbiturates by Heroin Addicts," *Canadian Medical Association Journal,* 98:1045–1049, 1968.

Davies, C., and S. Levine, "A Controlled Comparison of Nitrazepam ("Mogadon") with Sodium Amylobarbitone as a Sleep-Inducing Agent," *British Journal of Psychiatry,* 113: 1005, 1967.

deVries, H. A., and G. M. Adams, "Electromyographic Comparison of Single Doses of Exercise and Meprobamate as to Effect on Muscular Relaxation," *American Journal of Physical Medicine,* 51(3):130–141, 1972.

Essig, C. F., "Newer Sedative Drugs that can Cause States of Intoxication and Dependence of Barbiturate Type," *Journal of the American Medical Association,* 196:714–717, 1966.

Fort, J., "The Problem of Barbiturates in the United States of America," *Bulletin on Narcotics,* 16:17, 1964.

Gardner, A. J., "Withdrawal Fits in Barbiturate Addicts," *Lancet,* 1:337–338, 1967.

Goodnow, R. E., *et al.,* "Physiological Performance Following Hypnotic Doses of Barbiturates," *Journal of Pharmacology and Experimental Therapeutics,* 102:55, 1951.

Gupta, R. C., and J. Kofoed, "Toxicological Statistics for Barbiturates, Other Sedatives and Tranquilizers in Ontario," *Canadian Medical Association Journal,* 94:863, 1966.

Haider, I., "A Double-Blind Controlled Trial of a Non-Barbiturate Hypnotic—Nitrazepam," *British Journal of Psychiatry,* 114:337, 1968.

Hopf, H. C., *et al.,* "The Effect of Diazepam on Motor Nerves and Skeletal Muscle," *Journal of Neurology,* 204(4):255–262, 1973.

Jaffe, J. H., and S. K. Sharpless, "The Rapid Development of Physical Dependence on Barbiturates," *Journal of Pharmacology and Experimental Therapeutics,* 150:140–145, 1965.

Lader, M. H., and L. Wing, *Physiological Measures, Sedative Drugs, and Morbid Anxiety.* New York: Oxford University Press, 1966.

Landauer, A. A., *et al.,* "The Combined Effects of Alcohol and Amitriptyline on Skills Similar to Motor-Car Driving," *Science,* 163:467, 1969.

Matthew, H., *et al.,* "Nitrazepam—a Safe Hypnotic," *British Medical Journal,* 3:23, 1969.

Oswald, I., "Sleep, Dreaming, and Drugs," *Practitioner,* 200:854, 1968.

Rafoth, R., *et al.,* "The Effect of Diazepam on Physiologically Measured Stress," *Journal of Oral Surgery,* 33(3):189–191, 1975.

Stevenson, I. H., "The Effect of Chronic Barbitone Administration and Withdrawal on the Sensitivity of the Central Nervous System to Barbiturate," *British Journal of Pharmacology*, 37:502p–503p, 1969.

Whitlock, F. A., and J. E. Edwards, "Barbiturates in Impulsive Attempted Suicide," *British Medical Journal*, 1:443, 1967.

SEDATIVE TERMINOLOGY

Amytal	A barbiturate of intermediate action
Analgesic	A pain-relieving chemical
Around the turn	Having passed through the worst part of withdrawal
Barbs	Barbiturates
Blue heavens, blue angels	Amytal
Candy	Barbiturates
Cold turkey	Withdrawal without the tapering-off process
Coming down	The period when the effects of a drug begin to wear off
Double trouble	Tuinal
Downers	Barbiturates, tranquilizers, alcohol, depressants in general
Fruit salad	A game of taking many different pills
Goof ball	Barbiturate
Goofers	Doriden
Ludes	Quaalude
Miltown	Meprobamate, a tranquilizer
Nembies	Nembutal
OD	Overdose
O.T.C.	Over-the-counter drugs, nonprescription
Paper	Paper for writing prescriptions
P.G.	Paregoric
Phenos	Phenobarbital
Pink ladies	Seconal
Rainbows	Tuinal capsules
Red devils, red birds, or reds	Seconal
Seccy or seggy	Seconal
Tooies	Tuinal
Up	High on drugs
Wasted	Passed out from overintoxication
Yellow jackets	Nembutal capsules

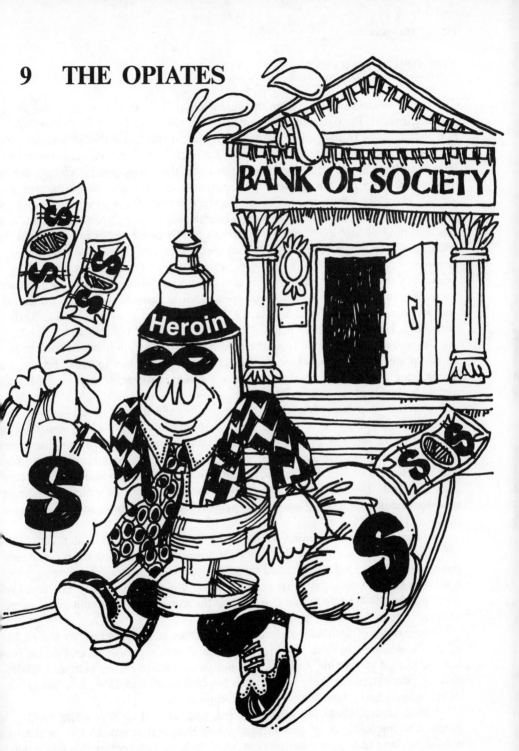

THE OPIUM HARVEST

The family of opiates derive from the parent plant *Papaver somniferum* and its raw exudate, opium. Poppy fields are planted in the fall or early spring throughout the belt that reaches from Turkey's Anatolian plateau through Pakistan and northern India to the "Golden Triangle" of Burma, Laos, and Thailand. About three months later the plants flower and, when the petals drop, the poppy pod is exposed. It is at this precise time (before the seed pod matures) that laborers score the pod in manner proscribed by centuries of ancestral experience. In Turkey the slashes are horizontal, in Southeast Asia they are vertical, while poppy growers in East Asia use a method of multiple scoring. The result of this procedure is the release of the white milky sap which oozes out, to be scraped off patiently by workers of the poppy fields within the next 24 hours. It is estimated that one person spends a full 40-hour work week to collect one pound of opium. The opium farmer in Turkey will receive about $60 for a kilo (2.2 pounds) of opium that is destined for heroin production (he will receive less, around $24 in 1972, if the opium is to be used for medical purposes). However, Turkey is not a large supplier of licit opium.

After opium is collected from the field it is air-dried until its water content is at an acceptable level for purchase. In this raw form it is brown in color, possesses a strong odor, and may be smoked, sniffed, or eaten; however, at this stage it is used mainly by locals of the cultivation areas.

The next step in processing is that of cooking out the rest of the water so that morphine content per unit weight rises to about 10%. By soaking and filtering opium with the addition of slaked lime and ammonium chloride, organic impurities are removed and morphine content rises to 50–70%. This is an intermediate product and not easily absorbed by the body; thus it is converted into morphine salt compounds or into heroin. The former of these two is the form in which morphine is used for medical purposes—morphine hydrochloride, morphine sulfate, and morphine acetate.

Diacetylmorphine is simply the morphine base that has been treated with acetic anhydride (or acetyl chloride, but since the former is less hazardous, it is the compound most often used) and passed through a process of heating and filtering which involves other chemicals such as acetone, alcohol, and tartaric acid. The resultant substance is called crude heroin and may be the same as No. 2 heroin in the heroin number code of Southeast Asia.

The natives of Southeast Asia use crude heroin to manufacture purple, or No. 3, heroin, which is smoked. The process is one of heating, crushing, and drying plus the addition of strychnine, caffeine, and barbitone (which offsets extreme intoxication), to the extent that heroin content is lowered to around 15%. It is tan to gray in appearance and granular or coarse in composition.

Crude heroin is also precipitated, dried, and crushed to form white, or No. 4, heroin, the injectable drug seen in the United States. It resembles talc or flour in consistency and may have a heroin content of 95% or more before it is adulterated.

ιe color varies from white to creamy yellow unless it comes from Mexico, in which
se its color is brown due to a chemical process differing from that used in Europe
ιd Asia.

After having been converted into one kilo of heroin, the original 10 kilograms
opium which was necessary to produce this amount of heroin is escalated in price
around $7000 in Marseilles. The border price for that same amount as it comes
ιo the United States rises to about $12,000, while the wholesale price in New York
ιty would be higher still—around $40,000. Finally, that amount sold on the street
ιuld go for over a quarter of a million dollars.

The escalation of price is due to the fact that great risks are involved and that
ιe heroin is cut, or adulterated, with milk sugar, quinine, mannite (a mild laxative),
ιd various other substances by all intermediate handlers until it averages anywhere
ιm 1 to 5% pure heroin on the street. The street user buys his drug in small lots—
"nickel bag" (five dollars' worth) which contains about 90 mg is enough to "get
ι." This is usually accomplished by liquifying the drug with tap water and "cook-
ι" it in a spoon or bottle cap, drawing it up through cotton into a 22- to 25-gauge
ιedle that has been affixed to an eyedropper, and then injecting it into a vein.

HE ECONOMY OF HEROIN ADDICTION

ιhe economics involved in the heroin addiction problem envelop monetary as well
ι social areas. Both can be explored for their cause and effect value, but only by
ιtimation. To begin to put a dollar value on heroin addiction in the United States,
ιe number of addicts and how much their habit costs per day must be known. With
conservative estimate of only 300,000 addicts, each with an average of a $60/day
ιbit, the cost of heroin alone is $18 million per day. It is well known that most
ιdicts cannot legally obtain the money required each day to support their habit;
ιus, if it is estimated that even 60% of addicts steal to provide money for heroin,
ιarly $11 million is still required daily. Since the return on stolen property is one
ιllar for every three to five dollars in value, the figure is escalated to 33 to 55
ιillion dollars per day of cost to the rest of society for heroin. Even the more
ιonservative figure of $33 million per day brings the total cost to society to 12
ιllion dollars a year.

In addition to the thefts, society pays for rehabilitation at an average of $1000
ι $3000 per year per addict, with approximately 100,000 addicts in some form of
ιeatment in 1974 [8].

This is only the financial aspect of the problem. The social aspects concerning
ιss in life quality and humanity to crime, prostitution, and the other dehumanizing
ιements of addiction cannot be measured except by a simple rate: one per addict.

Social statement must also be made concerning the nonaddict receivers of goods
ιtolen for drugs. Large cities such as New York may offer a greater opportunity for
ιhe addict to fence his stolen property, but sale of these goods has become an eco-

nomic institution in low-income areas. Taking advantage of cut-rate goods sto[l]
from the "Establishment" affords a feeling of "getting my share," even though it p[e]
petuates drug addiction in that very area.

PHARMACOLOGICAL EFFECTS

Heroin and the other opiates are narcotic sedatives that exert their effects by d[e]
pressing the central nervous system, especially the sensory areas of the thalamus a[nd]
cerebral cortex. This depressant action works to relieve pain and, in large doses,
induce sleep. Overdose causes death because of the narcotic's selective depressa[nt]
action on the respiratory center in the medulla.

Heroin has a rapid onset of action and proceeds with its analgesic effect. T[he]
results are a flush of euphoria, elevation of mood, and a feeling of peace, conten[t]
ment, and safety as the drug offers relief from the environment, both internal a[nd]
external. This is one of the most significant reasons why heroin has the highest addi[c]
tion potential of all the illicit drugs. Its analgesic effect is about three times that [of]
morphine—two to five mg of heroin via intramuscular injection has about the sam[e]
effect as 8 to 16 mg of morphine administered in the same manner or 300 to 6[00]
mg of opium given orally. Heroin is still used in Britain as a medicine and proves [to]
be an efficient tranquilizer, cough suppressant, and short-acting pain reliever. It al[so]
counteracts diarrhea and has been used in the treatment of cancer patients.

Common effects of the opiates (see Table 9.1) are respiratory depression (bo[th]
rate and depth), constipation, pupillary constriction, postural hypotension, libid[o]
suppression, and release of histamine (which causes the itching that may accompa[ny]
heroin use). Nausea and vomiting also often accompany heroin use, especially in th[e]
neophyte. Contrary to common belief, high-dose users of the opiates can functio[n]
quite adequately, and, aside from the danger of unsterile needles and other catastr[o]
phes due to the life-style of the heroin user, the addict does not suffer the physic[al]
deterioration caused by chronic use of other drugs such as alcohol. Diseases suc[h]
as hepatitis, septicemia, and endocarditis accompany the use of unsterile needle[s]

TABLE 9.1
Opiate drugs: their origin and potency

Drug	Origin	Potency
Laudanum	Alcoholic solution of 10% opium	0.10X opium
Paregoric	4% tincture of opium	0.04X opium
Morphine	Natural alkaloid	10X opium
Codeine	Natural alkaloid	0.50X opium
Heroin	Semisynthetic	3X morphin[e]
Dilaudid	Semisynthetic	3–4X morphin[e]
Meperidine	Semisynthetic	0.1X morphin[e]
Methadone	Synthetic	equals morphin[e]

d abscesses are common among heroin addicts, also. Another cause of fatality in roin addicts is cardiovascular collapse due to allergic reaction to the injected bstance.

Heroin's pharmacological action is that of morphine because it is converted ck into morphine in the body. Thus, both drugs are eliminated through the urine morphine, which becomes the basis of urinalysis. It is also eliminated in the east milk of a lactating mother, and in sweat and saliva. Because it easily crosses e placental barrier, infants born of addicts come into the world as narcotic addicts, o. They are given paregoric, tincture of opium, or methadone in decreasing dosage til the physical dependence is alleviated.

The adult addict's perils parallel the infant's need to allay withdrawal. As the fects of an injection of heroin wear off, the addict generally has four to six hours which to find his or her next supply. If a strong depressant is not taken within this ne, withdrawal symptoms begin to appear—runny nose, dilation of pupils, stom- h cramps, chills, and the other symptoms of the classic abstinence syndrome. Bar- turates, nonbarbiturate sedative hypnotics, cough syrup with codeine, or other ch depressants may be used by the addict to postpone withdrawal if heroin or the oney to purchase it is not available.

In cases of overdose, addicts are given narcotic antagonists such as levallorphan, alorphine, or naloxone that will reverse the acute, life-threatening respiratory de- ession. Using such antagonists counteracts the pharmacological action of narcotics d, in essence, induces "cold-turkey" withdrawal.

The addict's preferred form of administration of the opiates is intravenous be- use of the immediate rush that is felt. Experienced opiate addicts can discern eroin from morphine because its acetylated form assists its entry into the central ervous system. Other forms of administration include snorting (sniffing), intra- uscular injection (skin-popping or joy-popping, or as used in a hospital setting), nd smoking. Many of the American GIs who experienced heroin use in Vietnam noked it in tobacco cigarettes. The heroin used there was extremely more potent ian American street heroin because it was sold in almost pure form; but when noked, it was rapidly reduced in potency because the high burning temperature of e cigarette (around 850°C) destroys about 80% of the effect of the heroin [13]. hus, a milder dependence would form from smoking almost pure heroin than from ther modes of administration.

RADE ROUTES

our principal networks of opiate harvest and heroin production smuggle heroin into he United States [8]. The primary network is that of Turkey, France, Western Eu- ope, South America, Canada, and the United States. The second network involves he opium harvested in the "Golden Triangle" area of Burma, Thailand, and Laos. his travels through shipping points in Hong Kong, Malaysia, Bangkok, and the hilippines into Canada and the west coast of the United States.

The third network is that of India, Iran, Pakistan, and Afghanistan. The opiu of the latter two countries characteristically has a low morphine content and it a pears that this network is not a great contributor to the world's illicit heroin mark It should be noted here that India is the prime producer of licit opium (about 85' of total world exports of opium). About 90% of the opium produced for medici is used for morphine, most of which is converted into codeine. About 35% of li morphine is extracted from the crushed stems and pods (called poppy straw) of t plant. This is the most efficient way to produce morphine, since the whole proce can be mechanized [2].

Upon serious curtailment of the entry of French heroin into the United State Mexican brown heroin appeared on the American scene, thus completing the maj networks of illicit import (Fig. 9.1).

HISTORY OF THE OPIATES

Historically, opium and its derivatives have single-handedly generated the deep fea of addiction and the drug addict in American society. Although history has not co tributed an answer to our heroin problem, it can ease the understanding of how th problem developed. This understanding then might be instrumental in developing new and workable approach to our addiction problem.

The history of opium begins centuries before the birth of Christ (circa 350 B.C.) in the country of Sumeria (now Iraq) where opium was used to treat dysen tery. The Sumerians soon carried this drug to Egypt and Persia, and Portugues sailors carried it to India. In the 10th century, it found its way to China. Throughout this time it was taken orally, as medicine, and generally not abused; but in the 17t century the Western custom of smoking came to Asia and opium smoking becam popular. Abuse of the drug first occurred on a large scale in India during the 17t century, when the drinking of alcohol was forbidden. Opium smoking soon becam a Chinese custom and vice, in spite of governmental edicts against its use and sal Thus, when the East India Company of England monopolized the Indian opiur trade, China no longer asked for gold and silver in exchange for tea and silk—i return, they imported opium. In 1729 (when the emperor imposed an edict agains opium) China was importing around 15 tons of opium per year, but by 179 imports had reached nearly 400 tons, due mainly to the involvement of the Eas India Company.

The opium wars were fought in 1839 and 1856 because China wished to en force an 1800 edict that banned opium importation, and European countries (sup pliers of opium) fought with them for better trade conditions. As an outcome Chin

Fig. 9.1 Major opiate smuggling networks and routes: (1) Turkey, France, Wester Europe, South America, and the United States; (2) Burma, Thailand, Laos, Hong Kong Malaysia, Bangkok, Philippines, and the United States; (3) India, Iran, Pakistan, an Afghanistan; and (4) Mexico and the United States. ►

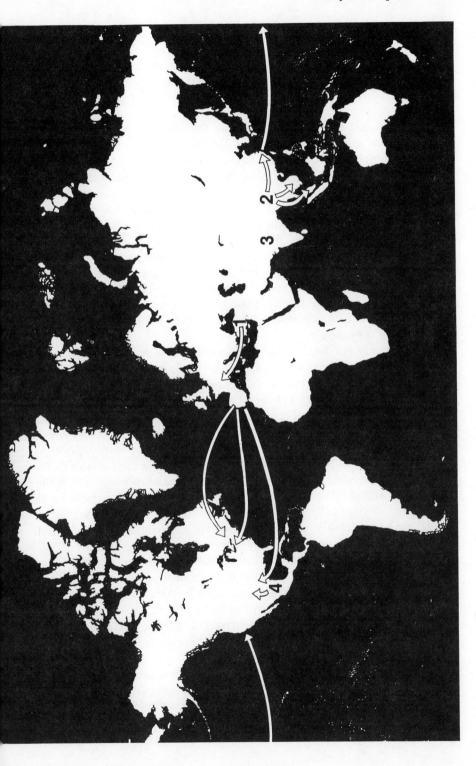

was economically forced to legalize the opium trade, a factor leading to widesprea
opium smoking and addiction.

From this series of events come the Chinese ancestors of America's opia
heritage. In the middle 1800s Chinese workers came to America to fill the lab
market for the railroad and canal projects that called for unskilled laborers. Wi
them came opium.

Its use caught on and opium became the analgesic property in many pate
medicines such as Dover's Powder or Dr. Barton's Brown Mixture. The opiu
derivative, morphine, was also heavily relied upon for treating wounded soldie
during the Civil War. During this time heroin was produced by the Bayer pharm
ceutical company in Germany and soon after was found to prevent withdrawal
morphine addiction, a condition that was present in about one out of 400 Amer
cans by the turn of the 20th century. Many soldiers exposed to morphine in the wa
continued their dependence, the general citizenry became dependent on the
favorite patented cure-all, and a limited number of individuals were abusing heroi

Except for a tariff imposed in 1842 on imported opium in order to regulate i
entry into the United States, the first step that the government took to regulate th
opiates was the passage of the Pure Food and Drug Act in 1906. This act demande
that all drugs containing opiates be labeled as such, so that consumers would kno
precisely what they were buying.

Growing concern for the addiction problem was made manifest in the time
honored tradition of the government: cut off the supply. This was attempted wit
the 1909 meeting of the International Opium Commission in Shanghai, at which th
United States pressed for such stringent control of opium production and trade tha
the other 12 countries present could not support the request. The goal of the Unite
States was total prohibition of opium in all countries in which it was cultivated, t
be effective immediately. Since many of these countries depended on opium export
in their balance of trade, the American position was less than tenable to them. Be
cause the 1909 meeting did not produce a treaty, the same group met in the Hagu
in 1911 and agreed that governments should control narcotics at both national an
international levels. In the United States the Harrison Narcotics Act naturally fol
lowed these international events; there is even speculation that these conferences wer
staged to persuade the passage of the Harrison Narcotics Act in 1914 [17].

Historically it appears that the United States was the only country strongly af
fected by the problems of addiction and throughout the Geneva Conference in 192
and 1925 all participating countries were urged by America to honor the agreemen
of the Hague Convention. It was obvious by this time that America could not con
trol its addiction problem and that the task entrusted to law enforcement had too
many ramifications to be simply treated with a total prohibition policy. Since the
Harrison Narcotics Act limited the legal supply of opiates to addicts, they had to g
"underground" to get their drugs. This is highly consequential, since it marked the
beginning of the illicit, street-drug culture that terrifies America today. Individua
physicians attempted to aid their addicted patients, but in 1915 the Treasury Depart
ment (in charge of enforcing the Harrison Narcotics Act) stated that physicians who
were treating narcotics addicts had to show decreasing doses over a period of time

oncompliance was considered violation of the Act. Subsequent court decisions against maintaining an addict, along with pressure on physicians from the American Medical Association Drug Committee to accept the police policy and stay out of the morphine-prescribing business, took most physicians out of the picture.

The government attempted to help addicts who were shut off from legal drug supply through the establishment of morphine clinics which opened in some of the large cities [24]. Here morphine was provided in order to curb antisocial behavior and to aid the addict in withdrawal from his or her drug habit, but crime rates rose as addicts from outlying areas came in droves to the city for free morphine, thus contributing to the poor living conditions already there. After several years all of these clinics had closed down in failure. They had not conquered the problem—in fact, addiction had increased.

The most intense addiction problems have characteristically been centered in large cities, especially those of the east and west coasts. New York City at present has the largest population of addicts and serves as a model of how the problem has progressed in the United States.

To take a small step backward, morphine or heroin addicts in New York City at the beginning of the 19th century were mostly people of the "nightlife"—prostitutes, pimps, and pickpockets—with the blacks, Jews, Irish, and Italians being the main ethnic groups involved. Other than the brief governmental effort to provide clinics to aid addicts in social recovery, society gave little attention to the addict throughout this period up through World War II, when heroin trade routes were interrupted and heroin use was at a standstill.

From about 1947 to 1951 heroin use began to spread rapidly through the large black and Puerto Rican and other low-income neighborhoods that had sprung up as a result of the influx of low-salaried workers into New York City during the war. Heroin was a dollar a "cap" (a No. 5 capsule, the smallest used by pharmaceutical companies), and sharing one's cap with two or three others was a common social occurrence. The heroin get-together of that era was probably much like the "pot party" of today so far as group oneness, ritual, and secrecy are concerned. Of deep social interest here is the fact that the addict could support his or her habit on a dollar or two a day; consequently, crime was not associated with heroin use as it is today. Another point of interest is that the typical heroin users of that time were employed workers in their twenties or thirties, not teenagers. However, around 1951 heroin use did start slipping down into the ranks of the teenager. Why this occurred is difficult to pinpoint, but the "cool" youth was no longer the leather-jacketed, fighting gang member, but rather the young heroin addict on the nod. Use by teenagers grew throughout New York City, and with this new drug-using population came a number of repercussions: (a) indignation that anyone could supply such a harmful drug to youngsters, (b) a rising crime rate, because these youngsters did not have jobs to provide for their habits, (c) increased publicity given to both the humanitarian and the crime aspects of the problem, and (d) increased prices put on the heroin itself because of the wider market and the bigger risk involved in selling to minors.

During this period organized crime, or the "syndicate," was the instrument for drug trade and other moneymaking operations such as loan sharking, bookmakin and the numbers game. But after the passage of the Narcotics Control Act in 195 which put very harsh penalties on violations of federal narcotic laws, and after a alleged split between older and younger groups within the syndicate [21], the olde established group withdrew from the heroin trade [3]. However, they loaned larg sums of money (at high interest rates) to the group still interested in the drug trad and thus still profited from the sale of heroin. It is said that the Mafia controls 80% of the U.S. heroin trade today [19].

In 1961 a shortage of heroin caused prices to soar, and as dealers of this na cotic realized that users would still buy low-quality heroin at high prices, the pric of heroin steadily increased. Now that an average user's habit cost more than $15 day, heroin addicts no longer tended to gather and share their magic powder; n longer could they keep up their normal family relationships; and no longer did ident fication with the addict culture serve as a social club membership. The life of th addict now became one of furtive, frequently criminal, effort to get his or her nex supply of heroin.

Of the estimated number of heroin addicts (which has ranged from 200,000 t 600,000 in the last decade), fully half of them are said to reside in New York, wit half of these living in New York City. This city bears its burden in many ways 50% of all crimes in New York City are attributed to the heroin problem and a estimated million dollars per day is lost in stolen property. Addiction is the greates single cause of death in the 15–35 age category and the age of addiction creeps lowe and lower.

In looking at this brief history of heroin use in New York City, we can see simi lar patterns developing all over the country. We can see why the alarm was sounde —once heroin use made its mark outside the low-income ghettos and began to present itself as a danger to the middle and upper-middle classes, the great cries o outrage were made. However, the country is still presented with the monumental tas of dealing with heroin addiction (and other drug abuse). In 1970 the Drug Abus Prevention and Control Act was passed, which for the first time provided a combi nation of prevention, treatment, and research, and also provided financial suppor for drug education in schools. In 1972 the Special Action Office for Drug Abus Prevention was created to strengthen prevention and rehabilitation efforts of the gov ernment. Effectiveness of this program is still to be tested, but it was a positive ste in treating the addiction problem, since a social dimension was added to law enforcement.

Although rehabilitation and prevention programs were instituted, the govern ment has persisted in its attack on illicit heroin entry into the country and its growth in foreign countries. In 1972 the United States paid Turkey 35 million dollars to stop growing the opium poppy and aided them in the cultivation of other agricultura crops. In 1974 Turkey decided that they would rather grow their old crop, that the United States should handle their opiate problem in ways that would not affec Turkish customs and economy. Also in 1974 the Drug Enforcement Administration (which grew out of the Bureau of Narcotics and Dangerous Drugs and other govern mental agencies involved in drug abuse) reported that the number of addicts had

ropped to about half the 1972 estimated number. DEA administrator John Bartels
tributed much of this to the breaking of the so-called "French Connection" through
e combined effort of American and French officials, but he attributed another part
f this decrease to methadone programs and to the addicts' switch to other drugs
hen European heroin became unavailable [26].

With a knowledge of the historical background of heroin abuse, it appears that
vo concurrent courses of action must be taken, that of *education* and that of *treat-
ent and rehabilitation,* if the problem of heroin addiction is to be dealt with
ffectively.

HE ADDICT

efore we can accomplish either education or treatment and rehabilitation (espe-
ially the latter) with satisfactory results, something must be known about the ad-
ict. One hears of the "addictive personality," but there is no study at this time that
ives any definitive information on preaddiction personality. Perhaps the addictive
ersonality that is so quickly offered as the cause of addiction is instead a *post-
addiction* personality—fearful, lacking self-assurance, criminal, psychotic, etc. There
s no simple explanation of what circumstances—social, chemical, physical, and psy-
hological—bring about addiction. Therefore, education must be aimed at all indi-
iduals, whereas treatment and rehabilitation must be directed toward the separate
ndividuals who have fallen into heroin addiction.

Even though the incidence of heroin addiction among white, middle-class,
ollege-age individuals is increasing, heroin addiction is still largely a problem of the
young, lower-class black or brown male [5]. In view of the fact that there is no
nherent strength genetically coded into the middle-class white and omitted in the
ower-class black, one might suggest sociopathology as the basic causative agent.
However, while the incidence of heroin addiction in the ghettos is epidemically high,
he majority of the population there does not use the drug. Thus we can conclude
generally that heroin addiction involves personality problems, but that these are
inseparable from social conditions.

Examining past histories of heroin addicts, Chein [4] describes not an addictive
personality *per se,* but an underdeveloped personality, one that is retarded in development by pathological social conditions. This may account for the high incidence
of drug experimentation in the ghettos. It is difficult to pinpoint the initial factor, but
the slums are basically places of high anxiety and frustration, with little development of competence to handle them. Broken homes are commonplace, and children
and parents all suffer the obvious disadvantages. Even in homes in which the parents
have managed to stay together, the fatigue and preoccupation with life struggles
allow little time for gaining insight into the child's role and human individualism.
Expectation, as well as discipline, is sporadic, based on mood. Goals are often unrealistic dreams. Graduating from this impoverished preschool environment, these
individuals are often seen as unteachable and incorrigible misfits by inexperienced

teachers. On the street, an aimless delinquent subculture develops as the only symp
thetic diversion to a hostile home and school environment.

Superficially, there is nothing mysterious or obscure about the conflicts th
develop in these situations, but researchers have been a bit overzealous in reasonir
that these conflicts are responsible for a lifelong desire to withdraw. More reali
tically, these may be powerful motivators for initial experimentation, for few exan
ples of consistent psychopathological personality have been observed when the dru
cycle has been blockaded in programs such as methadone maintenance [9].

Rehabilitation of the addict has not enjoyed a great deal of success in our cour
try, because the life of addiction has been a total life to the addict. Heroin is not ju
a chemical taken at intervals; it is a social life, a psychological life, a physical life–
in fact, the addict's life is totally centered around that necessary chemical. For exan
ple, imagine having an enormous appetite for food. Food is in your dreams an
daydreams. Now imagine that you eat whatever you like, whenever you like. Obesit
develops; but you still languish in food, you savor every bite. You must, legally o
illegally, provide money for food. You avoid normal-weight people, especiall
dieters. You enjoy dinner parties and other gatherings where there is food, and you
social life is contoured by this basic desire for food. When you are at work, yo
become anxious and "fidgety" before coffee breaks and lunch hour, and especiall
toward the end of the day when you can go home to a sumptuous meal and evenin,
snacks.

Now suppose your physician or your friends recommend that you go on a die
to lose those 100 extra pounds. Or perhaps you have a heart attack and *must* cu
down to a mere 500 calories a day!

If you can imagine yourself in this situation (or in that of giving up any desir
able habit), the position of the addict and his or her life of addiction become cleare
and the terms "treatment" and "rehabilitation" are made more vivid. For this obese
person (or anyone who finds he or she must diet or give up any other ingrainec
habit), food is not the only missing element—it is the *whole life built around eating*
that is missed. This person must fill his time with something other than eating; he
must alter his social pattern so as to exclude dinner parties or other gatherings where
caloric snacks are served; indeed, he must alter his whole life pattern to exclude all
his old eating habits.

In Fig. 9.2 we see the elements that combine to create obesity. Substitute heroin
(or some other drug) for food in this diagram, and we see the forces that create the
addict. In order to "cure" the addict, all of these forces must be remolded without
the drug. In everything the addict does, he or she has been conditioned for existence
in the drug world. Now he or she must be *reconditioned* so that the absence of the
drug does not leave a huge void. To the addict, only money and heroin count. In
the process of rehabilitation something must be substituted for heroin, and the first
step in this substitution is that of filling up time. Now the addict has all the time in
the world—time formerly spent in the cycle of hustling and shooting up. Now that
time must be filled with nondrug-oriented behavior, and unless supportive aid is
given, this sick, disoriented person who continually has the feeling that "something
is missing" will go back to the old drug life to fill up his or her time.

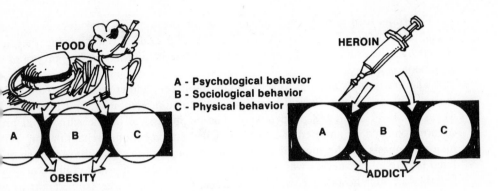

Figure 9.2

It is because of this need for multidimensional reorientation that only a small percentage of heroin addicts up to this time have been cured. Treatment and rehabilitation attempts must strive for this goal, and the closer they come, the higher the cure rate will be. With this in mind, we will look at the current treatments and rehabilitation programs available in the country today, and point out in what ways they serve the addict.

Since addiction to the opiates has existed for centuries, one might assume that knowledge of causative factors and methods of rehabilitation would be well advanced. Unfortunately, program after program has been theorized, tried, and shelved in the attempt to control addiction and the sociopathology surrounding it. The difficulty lies in the psychosocial components of addiction. Even though there are no preaddictive personality traits that can be used to predict which members of our society will become influenced and subsequently driven by heroin, there are any number of traits that are shared by the majority of heroin addicts. Reiteration of psychosocial traits of the addict, as reported by Chein *et al.* [5] in 1964 and continually validated by subsequent research, are given in Table 9.2.

TABLE 9.2
Psychosocial traits of the heroin addict

Social	Psychological
Lower-class black or brown male	Weakness of character
Impoverished	Self-indulgent quest for euphoria
Pathological social conditions	Need to escape reality
Broken homes	Emotional preoccupation with self
Poor parental guidance	Fearful
in discipline or goals	Lacking self-assurance, self-confidence
Poor family cohesiveness	Underdeveloped personality
Criminal	Retarded development
	Feeling of futility
	Feelings of negativism

The traits seen in Table 9.2 do not describe every addict, nor does every individual with many of these traits become a heroin addict. But knowing they are shared by a large number of our addicts should be helpful in devising programs of treatment.

The first serious attempt to rehabilitate the heroin addict became a reality with the opening of the two federal hospitals at Lexington, Kentucky, and Fort Worth, Texas, in 1936 and 1938, respectively. The emphasis was on the withdrawal procedure, followed by an attempt at psychological and vocational rehabilitation. With major emphasis on the medical aspect and minor emphasis on those traits as outlined in Table 9.2, success was not to be expected, and the absolute failure of these federal narcotics hospitals is well known. The return rate varies from report to report but approximately 95% of those treated eventually returned to drugs, 90% within six months after their release. Supporters of this program were quick to point out such obvious factors as forced confinement and quick release as major contributors to failure. Not denying that these built-in pitfalls were significant, one must also consider the methods and underlying philosophies of the program, which in retrospect seem to have been based more on legal detoxification than on psychosocial support. Being unable to rationalize the support of a heroin habit, hospital authorities gave primary consideration to abrupt and absolute withdrawal; thus, little attention was given to prewithdrawal support, sensitizing, or building of incentive.

The socially conscious and enlightened 1960s did produce many programs which, although still in the experimental stage, seem promising, for they are based on more realistic theories. Dole and Nyswander [10] have been responsible for the inception of several new programs based on drug maintenance, centering their rehabilitation efforts on the idea that the symptoms of the addictive personality are a *result* of the completely life-engrossing drug habit and not the *cause* of it [9]. In regard to the traits listed in Table 9.2, the theory of Dole and Nyswander (as a prototype for maintenance programs) is based on eradication of social factors that keep the addict down; while the "third-world" approach (with Synanon as the prototype) focuses more on the psychological aspects. The theory behind the type of rehabilitation exemplified by Synanon revolves around personality growth and the development of self-confidence, self-concept, and self-reliance. Each of these basic approaches is preceded, however, by medical treatment or withdrawal from heroin, which takes place before rehabilitation is attempted.

Withdrawal

Addicts can be withdrawn from heroin either abruptly, as in Synanon, or gradually, as in hospital settings. Since the drug is a depressant, the administration of another strong depressant, in diminishing doses over a period of seven to ten days, will accomplish the medical task. Street heroin in the United States has been "oversold" as to the severity of withdrawal that it causes; this fact makes the process of withdrawal less life-threatening than the D.T.'s or withdrawal from sedative hypnotics or tranquilizers.

MAINTENANCE PROGRAMS

Much research in medicine centers on identification of the cause of a disease, and subsequent elimination of the cause usually eliminates the problem. However, with heroin addiction, there are two basic areas with which one must deal. The first is a *psychosocial circle* of conditions and events leading to experimentation with heroin; the other is a *psychophysiological circle,* which necessitates continuation of heroin use. If all the psychological and social conditions mentioned earlier in this chapter were responsible for drug use, then we would have to rid the addict of these factors so that stronger, more adaptive personalities would develop. Although this is not a realistic short-range goal for our society, "third communities" such as Synanon are evidence that a change in environment will support drug abstinence.

Since American scientific technology has advanced more rapidly than have social conditions, it would appear that the psychophysiological circle would be the more profitable of the two on which to work, even if such work were only a stopgap measure. Programs based on this premise are called *maintenance programs.* Although they are now being used in many countries of the world, the program in use in England has received the most publicity and is known as the "British system." In this program, the addict receives a regular daily supply of opiates free or at minimal cost. He or she is under the supervision of a knowledgeable and ethical physician who supplies the addict's maintenance needs. The program is in the hands of a specialized individual in each area, thus reducing the corruption that once plagued the system. While the British have not legalized heroin possession, its use under a physician's care is legal. The drug culture there remains basically stable, and little crime is attributed to opiate addicts [17]. In this program the addict does not spend his life seeking sources of heroin or goods to pay for it.

Methadone maintenance

A similar system in the United States is the use of methadone maintenance. Methadone (diphenyl-dimethylaminoheplanone—trade and generic names include Methadone hydrochloride, Adanon HCl, Dolophine HCl, Althose HCl, and Amidone HCl), like morphine, is an analgesic drug, but is dissimilar in chemical structure. This completely synthetic substance does possess pharmacological characteristics much like those of morphine but has many practical advantages over the opiates [18]:

1. It can be taken orally, usually in 100-mg to 180-mg doses, mixed with drinks such as orange juice.

2. Its metabolism is sufficiently slow to prolong its action for 24 hours.

3. It is less likely to cause toxic side effects, such as the menstrual irregularities suffered by most female addicts, than is morphine.

4. Most important, it suppresses desire for heroin primarily by blocking heroin euphoria and abstinence symptoms.

Methadone is a narcotic, and does produce tolerance and physical dependenc (see Chapter 8 for theories regarding these two phenomena). Although the mecha nism of its action is poorly understood, the theories resemble those put forth fo morphine. One of these theories hypothesizes a selective depression of interneuron of the spinal cord and postganglionic neurons of the autonomic system. Although it primary involvement seems to be with the cholinergic system (the system of nerv fibers activated by acetylcholine), findings of both increases and decreases in acetyl choline obscure exact evidence of its depressive mechanisms [15]. Depression o selected reflexes indicates action on the spinal cord, decreases in respiration rate in dicate action on the medulla, and decreases in body temperature indicate action o the hypothalamus [20]. Involvement with the hypothalamic-pituitary-adrenal axi may be indicated by suppression of the release of ACTH (adrenocorticotropic hor mone, the pituitary hormone responsible for initiating the stress response in the body), and could be responsible, therefore, for generally suppressed stress reactions The suppressed production of sex hormones could also be responsible for the men strual problems of the female and the loss of libido experienced by both sexes, bu much more research needs to be conducted on this hypothesis [7].

Aside from constipation, which is really a small price to pay, patients have no shown any major ill effects from taking methadone. Both mental and neuromuscula functions appear to be normal. Patients perform well at jobs and in the classroom In fact, researchers have not been able to find a medical or psychological test, excep urinalysis, that can distinguish methadone patients from normal individuals.

In the methadone maintenance program the addict's cycle of hustle, fix, hustle, fix is broken and the search for drugs is ended. In essence, he or she is stabilized ir a state of blockade, between euphoria and withdrawal. Patients have shown that they soon begin to tolerate frustrating situations without feeling the hunger for heroin. Their dreams and conversations about drugs begin to subside and often, when busy, they even forget periodic medication [10].

Comparing Fig. 9.3 with the original diagram of addiction in Fig. 9.2 we see

A - Psychological behavior
B - Sociological behavior
C - Physical behavior
M - Methadone treatment

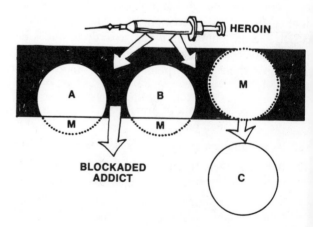

Figure 9.3

at methadone blocks the physical need for heroin, thus removing physical behavior from the heroin pattern. With this removal, changes in social and psychological behavior are evident, but depend solely on the maintenance drug. Unlike some f the self-help programs to be discussed later, methadone maintenance *per se* does ttle for psychological and social development. Indirectly, however, it does allow ddicts to stay off heroin, to get steady jobs, to support their families, and to get a tart on the way to becoming productive members of society. In this way methadone naintenance contributes not only to social factors, but to psychological factors as vell.

However, at this time there are a number of drawbacks to and criticisms of the methadone maintenance program:

1. Even though the daily cost to the addict is roughly that of a cup of coffee, the total treatment of each addict costs between $1500 and $2000 per year.

2. Doctors are justifiably reluctant to start young patients on a treatment that could keep them dependent for life.

3. It ties the addict to a daily ritual of receiving the medicine at outpatient clinics.

4. Methadone maintenance is at best an incomplete cure.

5. The giving of an addicting drug to drug addicts is contrary to our current morality.

6. Some methadone eventually finds its way into the street market.

One of these drawbacks is being eliminated through research on a newer substance, Acetylmethadol. This drug may help because it suppresses opiate withdrawal up to 72 hours and can be taken three times a week instead of seven, thus allowing more freedom for the patient [16].

Future research and enlightened attitudes may eliminate other drawbacks and even bring complete cure, but until then it makes little sense to withhold life-sustaining treatment from the afflicted. These individuals are caught up in the drug cycle now and cannot wait until the causative social and psychological conditions are eradicated.

Opiate antagonists

Other pharmacological substances have also been tried in an attempt to find a more practical pharmacological deterrent to heroin addiction. Nalorphine, Naloxone, and Cyclazocine are a few of the drugs classified as *opiate antagonists*. These are less objectionable than methadone from a moral standpoint, for they are antinarcotic and block the effects of morphine. Because of their toxic effects and their inability to relieve the craving for heroin, the antagonists are not as popular as methadone with patients. The mechanism of their action is not definitely known, but it is thought to be associated with increased acetylcholine levels at specific sites [14].

Treatment with Cyclazocine first necessitates withdrawal from heroin. Then Cyclazocine is administered in increasing doses until tolerance develops. The usual dose at which tolerance develops is about four mg per day. This level will block the subjective effects of 20 to 25 mg of heroin for a period of 20 to 26 hours. The addict is usually tranquil and free of anxiety, without any appearance of sedation or mental disturbance. Most important is the absence of the drive to find heroin, which allows for social rehabilitation and increased productivity.

Nalorphine is too short-acting to be of much clinical value; it is used more to detect the use of heroin and to counteract the effects of overdose. Naloxone must be administered in massive doses to achieve heroin blockage and since its supply is limited, its use is also limited. Still another substance of potential use in treating opiate addicts is being tested. This substance, Pentazocine, is an effective analgesic drug but, unlike the narcotic analgesics, it does not support morphine dependence. Many of the side effects attributable to Cyclazocine and Nalorphine are less severe with Pentazocine [6]. At this time there is very limited use of the antagonists in treatment programs because (1) they have unpleasant and disturbing side effects, (2) they must be administered daily, and (3) heroin addicts do not find these drugs helpful [25].

Synanon

Endore [12] has stated that society prepares the crime, while the criminal merely executes it; and goes on to say that Dederich, the founder of Synanon, has designed a new society for drug addicts in which they no longer *have* to be junkies.

Dederich, an ex-alcoholic, started Synanon on two basic assumptions: that the unadulterated truth was the only thing that could set addicts free, and that anything that was good for those who ran Synanon was good for all the individuals in Synanon. Thus addicts coming into Synanon were helped through "cold-turkey" withdrawal by ex-addicts, were given a job and money, and were forced to face the truth about themselves in their daily lives and in small-group encounters known as "synanons."

There are two basic rules at Synanon: no physical violence and no drugs of any kind. The addict is forced to conform or leave, because neither rule may be broken. If an individual wants to take drugs, he or she obviously must leave Synanon. Unlike hospitals, jails, or other institutions with which the addict may be familiar, there are no locks on the doors, and no guards at Synanon, so the addict can leave any time he or she wishes. To jail a person for taking drugs is to encapsulate the addict even more severely than he or she was encapsulated on the street in the world of drugs. Synanon works toward *un*encapsulating the addict.

A great deal is said about the small-group sessions in Synanon, but even its founder cannot fully explain them. They are dynamic encounters in which all the fury, frustration, and other deep emotions of one individual are pitted against all the others in the group. The only restraint is the basic rule of no physical violence. No one can hide from the truth, for other members turn their full vehemence on anyone who even appears to be deviating from the truth or hiding behind a lie. Since Synanon members live together within the organization's community, they relate with each other constantly, with all addicts learning more and more about themselves, others, and the nondrug life in general.

Addicts have been likened to little children who have not had a chance to mature or learn to live in a loving, caring, protecting world. Nearly every addict has lacked these qualities in his or her life, and at Synanon each is finally given the experience of knowing them. You cannot rule a child with punishment and hostility, because a child does not come into this world equipped with a sense of moral responsibility. To continually punish children for a reason that they do not understand is to place upon them a guilt for which they know no cause, and thus their development is arrested. At Synanon addicts are given the rest of their lives—if they wish to stay that long—to develop these missing characteristics. There is no one-year program, no five-year program, etc.—no specific time can be set on a cure for addiction. Some members move out of the Synanon community when they feel confident enough about their new nondrug life, but a large majority of the ex-addicts remain within the organization. This behavior reminds one of many small midwestern or southern towns of the past, in which most of the young people did not venture out into the world, but rather settled down in the same community to raise the next generation.

Thus Synanon offers a whole new society for the addict who is willing to give up his hate for life. He may come into this community of ex-addicts, get cleaned up, work, and rise to the top of the administrative strata if he wishes to assert himself. He is protected from his old life while he is reconditioned to a new life without drugs; he is lured into this new life by truth and by insight into himself.

Synanon has claimed the highest cure rate in any rehabilitation program to date [12]. Many people argue that this is due to the selective nature of the members who come into Synanon—people who voluntarily enter a program that they know will involve difficult problems of readjustment are obviously motivated toward cure—and perhaps this is an important variable. But the most important fact is that addicts have been transformed into complete human beings once again. This transformation has involved a change in all the factors of addiction—social, psychological, physical—and the chemical has been eliminated. We have seen that other treatment programs may attempt to change one or more of these factors, but unless all are ministered to, cure rates will continue to be low. The ex-addict must live a totally new life, totally different from the life of drugs or he or she may be led back to the drug by old drug-conditioned reflexes.

Through the aid of Synanon a completely new environment is substituted for the old heroin environment; thus our basic diagram of addiction can be revised to show all behavior moved outside of heroin into a new, drug-free world (see Fig. 9.4).

Halfway houses and other rehabilitation centers

There are other programs in the United States that offer the addict a place to reconstruct his or her life, but none appears to have the stability or the success of Synanon. The services offered by halfway houses range from the full-time residency, as at Daytop Village, to mere visits for counseling. These various programs throughout the nation are supported by a variety of institutions or organizations, and man-

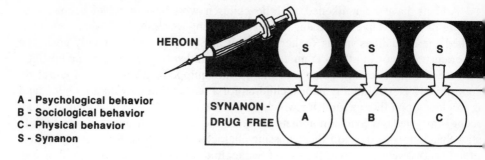

A - Psychological behavior
B - Sociological behavior
C - Physical behavior
S - Synanon

Figure 9.4

agement and philosophy differ from program to program. Most of these programs treat addicts who have come to them from the courts, and the program is designed to enable each addict to reenter society. Halfway houses will most likely enjoy limited success because of their inability to minister to all of the many factors that cause addiction.

Legislative programs

Civil commitment programs have been in existence in some states (led by California and New York) for about ten years. The primary purpose is to get the addict off the street and away from the public. In comparison with programs such as Synanon and methadone maintenance, which have had some measure of success in addict rehabilitation, these civil commitment programs may seem a step backward, but they are a temporary measure to protect society. Even if the heroin user is no more inherently criminal than anyone else, once on the heroin cycle his or her involvement with crime increases significantly. Alarcon [1] has clearly shown that one addict can be directly responsible for starting at least 30 additional users. Though all are not this prolific, most addicts are introduced to the drug by friends; thus, every one removed from the street reduces the number of potential addicts.

The particulars of these programs vary from state to state, but in general, when an addict is convicted of heroin addiction or of a civil crime while addicted, he or she may be sent to a rehabilitation center instead of prison [22, 23]. The systems have been notable for their inflexibility and some centers are considered little better than prisons, but the courts have realized the drug-compulsion motivation for the crime and often dismiss criminal charges after several years of successful parole [18].

In most cases the addict is sentenced to a definite period of time, which may vary from three to ten years depending on the offense. The first six months are spent in the rehabilitation center for withdrawal and determination of psychological and vocational aptitude. After a brief stay at a regional center, the individual is discharged on parole and is supervised as closely as possible. Some centers ask the parolee to report regularly to a clinic for Nalline tests. If he or she remains clean for the period of parole, he or she is discharged from commitment, and often criminal charges are completely dropped [11].

It is still too early to determine the effectiveness of the civil commitment pro-grams, but initial data reveal that only one in five addicts follows the above-mentioned pattern; the remainder spend about half of their sentence in confinement. Although the obvious benefactor is society, it seems that more emphasis on other successful programs would be of greater overall benefit, with less loss of personal freedom for the addict.

REFERENCES

1. Alarcon, R., "The Spread of Heroin Abuse in a Community," *Bulletin on Narcotics,* 21:17–22, 1969.

2. Cabinet Committee on International Narcotics Control, *World Opium Survey* 1972. Washington, D.C.: U.S. Government Printing Office, 1972.

3. Casey, J., Jr., "Taking Care of Business—the Heroin User's Life on the Street," *International Journal of the Addictions,* 4:1–24, 1969.

4. Chein, I., "Psychological, Social and Epidemiological Factors in Drug Addiction," in *Rehabilitating the Narcotic Addict.* Washington, D.C.: U.S. Department of Health, Education, and Welfare, 1967.

5. Chein, I., *The Road to H: Narcotics, Delinquency and Social Policy.* New York: Basic Books, 1964.

6. Collier, H. O. J., and C. Schneider, "Profiles of Activity in Rodents of Some Narcotic Antagonist Drugs," *Nature,* 224:610–612, 1969.

7. Cushman, P., *et al.,* "Hypothalamic-Pituitary-Adrenal Axis in Methadone-Treated Heroin Addicts," *Journal of Clinical Endocrinology,* 30:24–29, 1970.

8. Drug Enforcement Administration, *Fact Sheets.* Washington, D.C.: DEA, 1974.

9. Dole, V. P., and M. E. Nyswander, "Heroin Addiction—a Metabolic Disease," *Archives of Internal Medicine,* 120:19–24, 1967.

10. Dole, V. P., and M. E. Nyswander, "Narcotic Blockade," *Archives of Internal Medicine,* 118:204–209, 1966.

11. Eddy, N. B., "Current Trends in the Treatment of Drug Dependence and Drug Abuse," *Bulletin on Narcotics,* 22:1–9, 1970.

12. Endore, G., *Synanon.* Garden City, N.Y.: Doubleday, 1968.

13. Gay, G. R., and E. L. Way, "Pharmacology of the Opiate Narcotics," in D. E. Smith and G. R. Gay, eds., *It's So Good Don't Even Try It Once,* pp. 45–58. Englewood Cliffs, N.J.: Prentice-Hall, 1972.

14. Harris, L. S., "Central Neurohormonal Systems Involved with Narcotic Agonists and Antagonists," *Federation Proceedings, Federation of American Societies for Experimental Biology,* 29:23–32, 1970.

15. Howes, J. G., *et al.,* "Brain Acetylcholine and Analgesia," *Journal of Pharmacology and Experimental Therapeutics,* 169:22–28, 1969.

16. Jaffe, J. H., *et al.,* "Comparisons of Acetylmethadol and Methadone in the Treatment of Long-Term Heroin Users," *Journal of the American Medical Association,* 211:1834–1836, 1970.

17. Kramer, J. C., "A Brief History of Heroin Addiction in America," in D. E. Smith and G. R. Gay, eds., *It's So Good Don't Even Try It Once.* Englewood Cliffs, N.J.: Prentice-Hall, 1972.

18. Kramer, J. C., "New Directions in the Management of Opiate Dependence," *The New Physician,* 18:203–209, 1969.

19. Lingeman, R. R., *Drugs from A to Z: a Dictionary.* New York: McGraw-Hill, 1974.

20. Martin, W. R., "Analgesic and Antipyretic Drugs," in W. S. Root and F. G. Hofman, eds., *Physiological Pharmacology.* New York: Academic Press, 1963.

21. Maurer, D. W., and V. H. Vogel, *Narcotics and Narcotic Addiction.* Springfield, Ill.: Charles C. Thomas, 1967.

22. McGee, R. A., "New Approaches to Control and Treatment of Drug Abusers in California," in D. M. Wilner and G. G. Kassebaum, eds., *Narcotics.* New York: McGraw-Hill, 1965.

23. Meiselas, H., "The Narcotic Addiction Program of the New York State Department of Mental Hygiene," in D. M. Wilner and G. G. Kassebaum, eds., *Narcotics.* New York: McGraw-Hill, 1965.

24. National Clearinghouse for Drug Abuse Information, "Report Series: Heroin," 33(1), January, 1975.

25. Select Committee on Crime (House Report 92-678), *A National Research Program to Combat the Heroin Addiction Crisis.* Washington, D.C.: U.S. Government Printing Office, 1971.

26. *U.S. News and World Report,* "Interview with the Administrator," April 1, 1972.

SUGGESTED READING

AMA Council on Mental Health, "Management of Narcotic-Drug Dependence by High Dosage Methadone HCl Technique," *Journal of the American Medical Association,* 201: 956–957, 1967.

AMA Council on Mental Health and the National Academy of Sciences, "Narcotics and Medical Practice: Medical Use of Morphine and Morphine-like Drugs and Management of Persons Dependent on Them," *Journal of the American Medical Association,* 202: 209–212, 1967.

Bearman, David, and Mimi Sheridan, "Patterns of Heroin Distribution in a White Middle-Class College Community," *Journal of Psychedelic Drugs,* 4(2):65–70, 1971.

Blakeslee, Alton, *What You Should Know about Drugs and Narcotics.* New York: Associated Press, 1969.

Bourne, P. G., ed., *Addiction.* New York: Academic Press, 1974.

Caldwell, J., et al., "The Biochemical Pharmacology of Abused Drugs III. Cannabis, Opiates and Synthetic Narcotics," *Clinical Pharmacology and Therapeutics,* 16(6):989–1013, 1974.

Chein, I., et al., *The Road to H: Narcotics, Delinquency, and Social Policy.* New York: Basic Books, 1964.

Cherubin, G. E., "The Medical Sequelae of Narcotic Addiction," *Annals of Internal Medicine,* 67:23, 1967.

Duncan, T. L., *Understanding and Helping the Narcotic Addict.* New York: Prentice-Hall, 1965.

Eddy, N. B., H. Halbach, H. Isbell, and M. H. Seevers, "Drug Dependence: its Significance and Characteristics," *Bulletin of World Health Organization,* 32:721, 1965.

Edwards, C. W., *Drug Dependence: Social Regulation and Treatment Alternatives.* New York: J. Aronson, 1974.

National Conference on Methadone Treatment Proceedings. Washington, D.C.: Fifth National Conference on Methadone Treatment, March 17–19, 1973.

Gay, Anne C., and George R. Gay, "Haight-Ashbury: Evolution of a Drug Culture in a Decade of Mendacity," *Journal of Psychedelic Drugs,* 4(2):81–90, 1971.

Gould, L. C., *Connections; Notes from the Heroin World.* New Haven: Yale University Press, 1974.

Harms, E., *Drug Addiction in Youth.* Oxford: Pergamon Press, 1965.

Jaffee, Saul, *Narcotics: an American Plan.* New York: Hill and Wang, 1966.

Kramer, J. C., "New Direction in the Management of Opiate Dependence," *The New Physician,* 18:203, 1969.

Krantz, J. C., "The Fate of Heroin in Man," *Current Medical Dialog,* 39:296–297, 1972.

Kron, Yves J., *Mainline to Nowhere: the Making of a Heroin Addict.* New York: Pantheon, 1965.

Lerner, Steven E., R. L. Linder, and Irving Klompus, "The Cost of Heroin to the Addict and the Community," *Journal of Psychedelic Drugs,* 4(2):99–103, 1971.

Lindesmith, A. R., *Addiction and Opiates.* Chicago: Aldine, 1968.

Louria, D. B., R. Hensel, and J. Rose, "Major Medical Complications of Heroin Attraction," *Annals of Internal Medicine,* 67:1, 1967.

Maurer, D. W., and V. H. Vogel, *Narcotics and Narcotic Addiction.* Springfield, Ill.: Charles C. Thomas, 1967.

National Conference on Methadone Treatment Proceedings. Washington, D.C.: Fifth National Conference on Methadone Treatment, March 17–19, 1973.

O'Donnell, John A., and John C. Ball, eds., *Narcotic Addiction.* New York: Harper & Row, 1966.

Pearson, J., *et al.,* "The Neuropathology of Heroin Addiction," *Journal of Neuropathology and Experimental Neurology,* 31:165–166, 1972.

Pittel, Stephen M., "Psychological Aspects of Heroin and Other Drug Dependence," *Journal of Psychedelic Drugs,* 4(2):40–45, 1971.

Rosenstein, B. J., "Viral Hepatitis in Narcotic Users," *Journal of the American Medical Association,* 2:3–20, 1967.

Smith, D. E., and G. R. Gay, *It's So Good Don't Even Try It Once.* Englewood Cliffs, N.J.: Prentice-Hall, 1972.

Taylor, N., *Narcotics: Nature's Dangerous Gifts.* New York: Dell, 1966.

Taylor, S. T., M. Wilbur, and R. Osnos, "The Wives of Drug Addicts," *American Journal of Psychiatry,* 125:585–591, 1966.

Vaillant, G. E., "A Twelve-Year Follow-Up of New York Narcotic Addicts: I. The Rela tion of Treatment to Outcome," *American Journal of Psychiatry,* January 1966 and November 1966.

VanVunakis, Helen, *et al.,* "Specificities of Antibodies to Morphine," *Journal of Phar macology and Experimental Therapeutics,* 180:514–521, 1972.

"Viet Heroin Abuse Drops but Problem Still Severe," *Journal of the American Medica Association,* 219:1280–1281, 1972.

Weech, A. D., Jr., "The Narcotics Addict and 'The Street'," *Archives of General Psy chiatry,* 14:299, 1966.

Wikler, Abraham, *et al.,* "Limbic System and Opioid Addiction in the Rat," *Transactions of the American Neurological Association,* 96:328, 1971.

Wilner, D. M., and G. G. Kassebaum, eds., *Narcotics.* New York: McGraw-Hill, 1965.

Yerby, A. S., "Problems of Neonatal Narcotic Addiction," *New York State Journal of Medicine,* May 15, 1966.

OPIATE TERMINOLOGY

Analgesic	Pain-relieving chemical
Around the turn	Having passed through the worst part of withdrawal
Artillery	Outfit for injecting drugs
Bag	Small quantity of drugs
Bagman	Small-time drug supplier
Bamboo	Opium pipe
Belly habit	Opiate addiction (first signs of withdrawal are stomach cramps)
Big man	High-level pusher
Burned out	Sclerosis of veins from puncturing
Cap	Capsule of drug
Coast	Euphoric nodding state of the heroin high
Cold turkey	Withdrawal without the tapering-off process
Cooker	Spoon or bottle cap to mix and heat heroin for injection
Cut	Dilute drugs, usually with milk sugar
Dabble	Use drugs irregularly
Dealer	Seller or pusher of drugs
Dried out	Withdrawn from drugs completely
Dynamite	High-grade heroin, sometimes mixed with cocaine
Fix	A shot of narcotics
Flash	Sudden rush or euphoric feeling
Flea powder	Inferior or phony drugs
Glow	High, euphoria

H	Heroin
Hard stuff	Opiates, heroin
Hooked	Addicted
Horse	Heroin
Jones	Heroin withdrawal
Joy-pop or skin-pop	Inject drugs under the skin
Junk	Narcotics
Junkie	One who uses narcotics regularly, usually addicted
Kick	Break the drug habit
Lemonade	Poor-grade heroin
M	Morphine
Mainline	Inject drugs into a vein
Maintaining	Keeping a certain level of drug habit
Nalline	A semisynthetic derivative of morphine, Nalorphine hydro-chloride
Nickel bag	$5 worth of drugs
O	Opium
OD	Overdose
On	On drugs, under the influence of drugs
On the street	Out of jail
Putting the bean	Begging for narcotics
Scag	Heroin
Scars	Needle marks
Score	Find and buy drugs
Shoot up	Inject drugs
Shooting gallery	A safe place to shoot up
Smack	Heroin
Source	Steady supplier of drugs
Strung out	Being addicted
Taste	Small amount of drugs
Turned off	Withdrawn from drugs

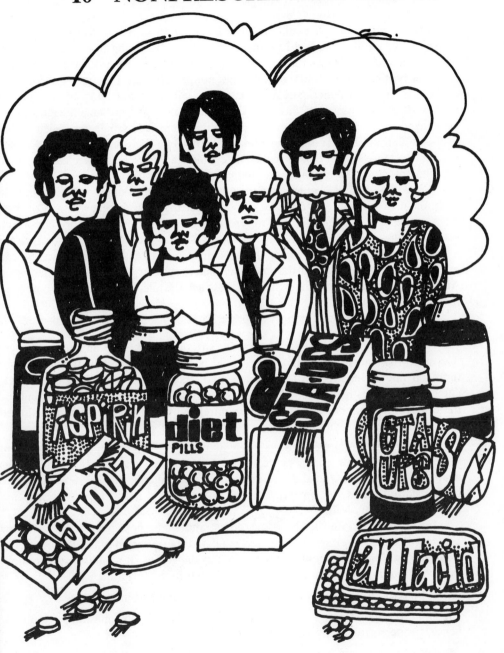

Americans are basically independent and like to take care of themselves, and professional medical care is rapidly pricing itself out of the reach of the majority of our population. The persuasive television announcer outlines symptoms and assures you that you are not alone, that millions have insomnia or simple nervous tension, and either can be easily remedied by simply, inexpensively, taking brand X or Y or Z. Thus the foundation is laid for a rapidly expanding multimillion-dollar industry that produces virtually thousands of different nonprescription (or over-the-counter) drugs. It is not that Americans have that many ailments, but hundreds of millions of dollars in advertisements have convinced us we do. We are encouraged toward self-diagnosis and self-medication for everything from falling hair and fallen arches to the condition of one's breath, stomach, or bowels. We are so convinced of the need for self-medication that in the average American household there can be found 30 different drugs, 24 of which are nonprescription.

While the average American does not buy over-the-counter (OTC) drugs in the pursuit of pleasure, he does seek and expect the drug to relieve some of life's painful reality. It is often said that we are a drug-using society, but more important, we are a drug-*mis*using society. If you define misuse as the taking of a substance for a purpose other than that which the substance was intended to produce or can produce, then you must add the multitudinous proprietary medicines to the list of America's misused drugs, the same list that includes alcohol, cigarettes, amphetamines, and barbiturates.

How can the taking of nonprescription drugs be justifiably labeled misuse?

1. Nonprescription drugs, for the most part, are ineffective and almost never live up to their advertising claims. It should be noted that the advertising is based more on underlying wants, needs, fears, and desires to escape, than on medical cures. Senate investigations over the last seven years have been looking not only at basic misrepresentation, but at the often unrelated psychological "gimmicks" used to promote these products.

2. Nonprescription drugs can be quite dangerous. There are dangers inherent in the chemical itself: dangers presented by personal idiosyncrasies (numerous deaths of individuals who did not know they were allergic to the substance have been reported), and the potential dangers of any drug used by persons who are unqualified to handle it.

Ineffectiveness often leads to overdoses, and since most people are somehow convinced that all dangerous drugs are regulated by prescription, they do not consider an overdose of a nonprescription drug as dangerous. It should be pointed out that only the *most* dangerous drugs are regulated by prescription.

3. Nonprescription drugs are diversions of both time and money.

4. Nonprescription drugs give a false sense of security by masking symptoms; hence, proper medical aid is not sought.

5. Perhaps the most important factor is that the "better things for better living through chemistry" idea is extended into the notion that there is a chemical cure-all for everything. This could be at the very root of America's drug problem.

This chapter presents only a few of the many classes of over-the-counter drugs, but this discussion should serve as a model to be applied to the overwhelming majority of other drugs that should be approached with extreme caution.

SLEEP AIDS

Most of the over-the-counter sleep aids are combinations of belladonna alkaloids and antihistamines (Table 10.1), and a number also contain salicylamide. The action of these substances is derived primarily from their anticholinergic properties (that is, they block acetylcholine at nerve synapses).

The effects of the anticholinergic agents are variable, unpredictable, and are often a bizarre combination of excitation and depression of the central nervous system. Most brands contain some combination of all three substances mentioned, and this often compounds the confusing symptomatology (Table 10.2) [12].

The *antihistamines* are commonly used to treat allergies and symptoms of the common cold (as the name implies, antihistamines block the vasodilation action that histamine exerts on the capillaries, thus decreasing fluid loss and congestion in the nasal cavity). The drowsiness or hypnotic side effects were, in the past, considered undesirable; today, it is the side effect that is being marketed!

The *belladonna alkaloids,* found throughout the world, are derivatives of the

TABLE 10.1
Ingredients of some common over-the-counter sleep aids and tranquilizers [5]

Sleep aid	Methapyrilene hydrochloride	Scopolamine hydrobromide	Salicyamide	Other
Nytol	25 mg			
Quiet Nite	25 mg			Phenylephrine Hydrochloride
Real Sleep	50 mg			Hyoscine hydro-
Sleep Aid	25 mg			bromide
Sleep Eze	25 mg	0.125 mg		
Sleep Tabs	25 mg	0.200 mg	250 mg	
Sominex				
Tablet	25 mg	0.250 mg	200 mg	
Capsule	50 mg	0.500 mg	200 mg	
Tranquilizer				
Compoz	15 mg	0.15 mg		
Quietran	12 mg	0.15 mg	325 mg	Acetophenetiden Thiamin
Tranqets	25 mg		250 mg	Ascorbic acid
Tranquizine	20 mg	0.10 mg	130 mg	Passiflora incannata Thiamin

TABLE 10.2
Summary of common effects from ingredients in popular OTC drugs [3, 5, 12]

Ingredients	Observed reactions from average dose	Observed reactions from excessive doses
Belladonna alkaloids		
Scopolamine*	Drowsiness	Dilated pupils
Homatropine	Euphoria	Flushed face
Atropine	Amnesia	Blurred vision
	Dreamless sleep	Somnolence
	Dry mouth	Restlessness
		Agitation
		Auditory hallucinations
		Visual hallucinations
		Delirium
Antihistamines		
Methapyrilene HCl *	Drowsiness	Blurred vision
Dipherhydramine	Lethargy	Nausea
Pheniramine	Dry mouth	Anxiety
Brompheriramine	Nausea	Vomiting
	Constipation	Tremors
	Dizziness	Delirium
		Convulsions
Salicylic acid		
Acetylsalicylic acid (aspirin)	Antipyresis	Nausea
Methyl salicylate	Analgesia	Dizziness
Salicylamide†	CNS depression	Emesis
	Anti-inflammation	Irritability
	Increased fecal blood	Dehydration
		Hallucination
		Convulsions

* Type most often used.
† Not metabolized as salicylate, but usually considered in this class.

plants of the nightshade or *Solonaceae* family. These substances can be classified as nonbarbiturate hypnotic sedatives. Their action of blocking acetylcholine or some peripheral cholinergic receptors has made them popular as involuntary muscle relaxants. In the Middle Ages they were the base ingredient of very popular poisons and were used for centuries in religious and magical rites. More recently, they have been used as a pre-anesthetic tranquilizer and as an antispasmodic for gastrointestinal disorders. In combination with the antihistamines, they often produce sedation. However, just as often, sedation is not produced! In view of the misuse of OTC sleep aids by the public, the best statement that can be made is that at recommended dosages they are often ineffective [12].

A recent study comparing one of the fastest-selling OTC sleep aids (containing 25 mg of methapyrilene and 0.25 mg of scopolamine, given at recommended dosages) with sugar cornstarch placebos led to the conclusion that the OTC sleep aids were no more effective than placebos in promoting or maintaining sleep [7].

Another study that produced similar results led to the conclusion that although the drug was limited in its effectiveness, many individuals will get sleepy after taking any pill that is represented to them as a sleep aid [9, 10]. Such is the power of advertising. Dr. C. Edwards of the Federal Food and Drug commission has estimated that 30% to 70% of any group of everyday people will respond to sugar pills if they are led to believe that they will be effective [13].

The over-the-counter sleep aids seem to the public to be a safe alternative to the prescription barbiturates. However, their effectiveness is doubtful and they too can be dangerous. Even in small doses, methapyrilene can produce side effects such as dizziness, blurred vision, dryness of the mouth, headache, ringing in the ears, and irritation of the digestive tract. Some people are affected in reverse, experiencing nervousness, tremors, restlessness, and euphoria [5]. Numerous clinical disturbances have been observed, and it has been noted by the manufacturers that glaucoma may be precipitated, especially in elderly people.

One problem inherent in the ineffectiveness of the OTC sleep aids is that when they do not give the desired results, users tend to overmedicate themselves. Two or three times the recommended dose has produced disorientation and hallucinations. Ullman [14], a London physician, suggests that it may be difficult to distinguish between toxic psychosis caused by OTC sleeping medications and acute schizophrenic reaction. Within one month he saw four patients suffering from hallucinations and delusions, three of whom showed methapyrilene in their urinalysis.

There have been several reported cases of attempted suicides with OTC sleep aids. These purposeful and extreme overdoses produced extreme confusion, psychiatric disturbances, a stuporous state, and coma. Deaths have also been reported [2].

Shader et al. [12] have identified at least 28 sleep-inducing medications that are available without prescription and contain, on the average, 0.125 to 0.5 mg of scopolamine. They suggest that these substances can produce euphoria and hallucinations, and represent an easily accessible, inexpensive, and legal source of intoxicants for pleasure-seeking youths.

The belladonna alkaloids are also the primary ingredient in medicines used to treat gastrointestinal maladies (they are included in a large number of laxatives), motion sickness, asthma (only recently a number of abused anticholinergic inhalants have been brought under the protection of prescription), eye conditions (in eye drops, they have led to a number of poisonings among children), and menstrual pain.

TRANQUILIZERS

Americans have become aware of and, to some extent, preoccupied with the detrimental effects of arousal caused by the stress and tension of modern society. It has been estimated that as many as one-half of the patients crowded into physicians' waiting rooms have ailments that either are entirely emotional or have significant emotional overtones. Consequently, tranquilizers rank just behind antibiotics as the most-often prescribed drugs. Capitalizing on this real or imagined need to diminish responsiveness to environmental and social stimuli, pharmaceutical manufacturers have marketed OTC products advertised as tranquilizers. The active ingredients are the same as those contained in the sleep-aid preparations, only in smaller doses and usually in combination with aspirin (see Table 10.1).

It should be recalled from the chapter on sedatives that tranquilizers are not just milder doses of the same ingredient found in the sedative hypnotics, such as barbiturates. They are different chemical substances with a different pharmacological action, and prescribed for different medical conditions. Even if the OTC sleep aids were effective, lesser amounts of the same product would produce sedation, which is an entirely different phenomenon from that produced by tranquilizers.

After studying the effect of OTC tranquilizers (Compoz), prescription tranquilizers (Librium), and a sugar pill placebo on patients showing mild to moderate symptoms of anxiety and tension, Rickels et al. (11) concluded that in terms of clinical efficiency, Compoz did not differ from the placebo. The prescription tranquilizers proved most effective, with no difference being observed between the OTC tranquilizer and the placebo. The patient who took a placebo, thinking it had therapeutic effects, did about as well as those who took the OTC tranquilizer, thinking it had therapeutic effectiveness.

ANALGESICS

It should come as no surprise that the most common analgesic in the world is aspirin (acetylsalicylic acid). Although this acid was not synthesized as aspirin until the nineteenth century, natural sources of its active ingredients have been used for thousands of years. Thanks to the stress and strain of our modern society (or to effective advertising), the "ailing" United States population's daily ingestion of aspirin tablets is rapidly approaching 50 million. There are hundreds of products that have acetylsalicylic acid as their primary ingredient (Table 10.3). Pharmaceutical manufacturers have buffered it, colored it, sugar-coated it; they have made it fizz, given it a round or oblong shape, and put it in time-release capsules. As the packaging changes, so does its use. One shape is advertised for use on the good old-fashioned headache; another shape for nervous tension. Of course, the ones for nervous tension caused by screaming children are different from the ones for nervous tension caused by missing a bus! If it is pretty enough and has a feminine-sounding name, women can use it for menstrual pain; and if it is candy-coated, children will enjoy it. Symptoms such as headache, upset stomach, and nausea constitute to millions of Americans a signal for the ingestion of aspirin. If one is looking for an example of drug misuse, aspirin consumption in the United States today would be as good an example as any.

TABLE 10.3
Ingredients in some popular OTC analgesics and antacids [3, 5]

Product	Aspirin	Caffeine	Magnesium hydroxide	Aluminum hydroxide	Other
Alka-Plus	X		X	X	Belladonna leaves
Aspergum	X				
Anacin	X	X			
Bufferin	X			X	Magnesium car- bonate
Chaser	X	X	X		Acetaminephen, Vitamin B
Co-Gel			X	X	
Cope	X	X	X	X	Methapyrilene fumanate
Excedrin	X	X			N-acetyl-p- ammophenol Salicylamide
Maalox			X	X	
Measurin	X				
Midol	X	X			
Mylanta			X	X	Semethicone
Standback	X	X			Salicylamide

Acetylsalicylic acid is truly a wonder drug. Its adverse effects are minimal compared to its beneficial pharmacological action. Still, aspirin follows only barbiturates, alcohol, and carbon monoxide in the number of fatal poisonings due to it annually. Excess use of aspirin has also been linked with certain kinds of kidney disease. Approximately two out of every 1000 persons are hypersensitive to aspirin and approximately 16% of asthmatic patients are allergic to it. Young children whose systems cannot withstand the dehydration and acid-base change are most affected. It should come as no surprise that the flavored compounds are responsible for 62% of the salicylate poisonings [3]. Another drawback to the use of aspirin has been reported by Dr. M. G. Blinder of San Francisco [8]. He has pointed out that since two aspirins can have an adverse effect on blood-clotting time for up to two weeks, women who use them immediately before or during their menstrual periods may double the blood volume lost, thus adding to their menstrual problems. Likewise, aspirin should not be taken before surgery or by a blood donor before giving blood. One of the more publicized dangers of aspirin, especially nonbuffered aspirin, is gastrointestinal bleeding which may result.

The effectiveness of aspirin in alleviating the pain of a headache is questionable and its use is definitely contraindicated with an upset stomach. An alternative might be another analgesic such as acetaminophen (the post popular source is the OTC analgesic, Tylenol). Acetaminophen, like aspirin, is reported to have analgesic and antipyretic action, but seems to be less toxic to the gastrointestinal system, resulting in less gastric blood loss, and does not seem to affect blood coagulation. Acetamino-

phen is not without potentially harmful side effects and Tylenol's label warn
against its use beyond 10 days. Of course, any symptom lasting that long shoulc
be brought to the attention of a physician.

Administration and absorption of aspirin

The rapid absorption of aspirin from the gastrointestinal tract is one of its most attractive features. Fifty percent of the normal dose of 650 mg (usually two 325-mg tablets) is absorbed within 30 minutes. The convenience of analgesia over an eight-hour period has prompted many pharmaceutical houses to develop time-release capsules. It was noted in one recent study, however, that the convenience of the time-release capsule may be overshadowed by decreased effectiveness. In a comparison of aspirin and Bufferin with Measurin, it was found that both aspirin and Bufferin produced higher early concentrations of salicylate and unhydrolyzed acetylsalicylic acid. The equal disappearance rate of the unhydrolyzed acetylsalicylic acid in the three casts some doubt on the benefits of prolonged-action preparations [6].

Primary pharmacological effects

Analgesic action. Empirical evidence would seem to indicate that acetylsalicylic acid is effective in the relief of pain. The evidence is still empirical, for researchers have not developed quantitative measures of pain relief or pain. Pain produced by pricking the skin, applying heat to the skin and teeth, sending electric current through metal dental fillings, etc., has produced conflicting results. Some studies have shown aspirin to be more effective than morphine and codeine [1], while others show aspirin as no more effective than a placebo.

There is still some controversy as to the site of the analgesic action of aspirin. Some researchers feel it is central in the hypothalamus, while others feel the action is peripheral. Still others believe the action to be purely psychological (the placebo effect).

It bears mentioning that even though the advertisements insinuate that aspirin will relieve the pain of a headache, they do not state this fact directly, for there is no evidence to support such a claim. Even though headache is the most "popular" ailment in the United States, not a great deal is known about its causes and cures. It would stand to reason that the most common type of headache, the tension headache, thought to be caused by the pain of tense muscles of the head and neck being referred to subcutaneous pain receptors around the head, would be predominant in fast-paced technological societies. Not all headaches are psychological, just most of them. Many are psychosomatic—the pain is as real as that caused by muscle tension. These headaches perhaps result from psychological stress and worry for which aspirin may offer some relief by dulling the perception of the pain. In Africa, Asia, and the Antarctic, headache is almost completely unknown. In industrialized South America and Europe, headaches are a minor nuisance of life and are not the topic of conversation, a convenient excuse, or an indication that the individual is important enough to have something to worry about. In the United States, however, advertising has elevated the headache to a national institution. Symptoms are outlined, throbbing pain is vividly described, and, most importantly, the social situations that might cause a headache are mentioned continually. An artificial ailment can usually be cured by a substance that is *perceived* as being effective. It is little wonder that 40% of each dollar spent on such products is spent on advertising.

Antipyretic (anti-fever) action. Infectious disease often causes the body to produce and contain increased amounts of heat. Body 'heat is elevated by increasing body metabolism and through muscular activity, usually shivering. The delicate temperature regulator, or thermostat, in the hypothalamus, although functional, becomes set at a higher level. Body temperature in relation to the thermostat is cool; thus, shivering is initiated while heat dissipation processes are decreased.

Although the exact pharmacological mechanism is not well understood, aspirin seems to lower the thermostat and allow for dissipation of heat through normal processes, such as dilation of cutaneous vessels. Aspirin is effective in the treatment of fever, but it will not lower temperature in individuals with normal body temperature.

Anti-inflammatory action. Acetylsalicylic acid has become one of the most-used therapeutic agents in the treatment of rheumatoid arthritis. Neither the pharmacology nor the mechanism of action is known, but aspirin seems to be effective in reducing the inflammation by decreasing the leakage of fluid from capillaries in the inflamed sac directly, or indirectly by action on the anti-inflammatory hormones produced by the adrenal cortex. Aspirin has also been shown to reduce fever associated with rheumatoid arthritis and to raise the pain threshhold by interfering with the brain's interpretation of the pain or through interference with peripheral transmission [3].

STIMULANTS AND ANTIOBESITY PREPARATIONS

A large section of Chapter 6 was dedicated to showing that antiobesity preparations containing various amphetamines, while pharmacologically effective in curbing appetite, were not effective in long-term weight control. One could hardly expect nonprescription commercial preparations to be more effective! The "active" ingredients of these drugs range from caffeine and methylcellulose to various bizarre combinations of belladonna extracts, aconite root, and gelsemium.

Antiobesity preparations can be divided into the following categories:

1. *Bulk preparations.* These add bulk to the gastrointestinal tract for the purpose of producing a sensation of being filled. The active ingredient is usually methylcellulose, a nonabsorbable cellulose that is supposed to swell in the stomach. Popular examples of this type of preparation are: Melozets, containing methylcellulose, flour, and sugar; Metamucil, containing dextrose, psyllium, and muccilloid; and Reducets, containing methylcellulose.

2. *Low-calorie foods and artificial sweeteners.* These are sold as drugs in drugstores and as food in supermarkets, but probably should be best classified as a food.

The most popular example in this category is Metrecal, which contains dry milk, soy flour, sugar, starch, dried yeast, corn oil, coconut oil, and vitamins.

3. *Benzocaine preparations.* These are substances that act as local anesthetics to diminish response and sensitivity of the stomach. Examples of this type are Shape Up, containing benzocaine and sodium carboxymethylcellulose, and, Slim Mint, which contains benzocaine, methylcellulose, and dextrose.

4. *Glucose preparations.* These substances use glucose to stimulate the satiety centers of the hypothalamus, thus reducing physiological hunger. Examples here are Ayds, which contain corn syrup, vegetable oil, vitamins, and sweetened condensed whole milk; and Proslim, which contains soy isolate, sucrose, dextrose; and powdered milk.

The active ingredient in most OTC stimulants is caffeine, a derivative of xanthine, and indigenous to coffee, tea, and many soft drinks (especially the colas). Caffeine does produce some stimulation of the central nervous system, and in most individuals will result in slight wakefulness, restlessness, and mild excitement. Although the diuretic action may promote dehydration, most normal individuals will not be harmed by it. Popular examples are Vivarin (200 mg of caffeine per tablet) and NoDoz (100 mg of caffeine per tablet). Excess caffeine may be contraindicated in persons with heart disease.

OTHER OVERUSED "MEDICINES"

Antacids, laxatives, and acne preparations are all becoming extremely profitable products for pharmaceutical companies. Although they basically do what they are intended to do, these preparations are much overused. Worry about regularity, like worry about not being able to sleep, is probably the greatest cause of the problem. More harm is usually done by attempts at chemical regulation than by the malady itself.

Americans spend well over 100 million dollars annually on antacid preparations. They come in every conceivable size, shape, and form to fit the needs and convenience of the users. There are over 300 different brands of tablets, pills, gums, and lozenges, about 150 liquids, and over 100 different powders.

Active ingredients in the nonabsorbable antacids are usually combinations of magnesium and aluminum hydroxide, but a wide variety of ingredients may be encountered (see Table 10.3). Antacids are usually considered effective if used properly; however, overuse can cause problems. Many of these preparations use aspirin and, as was previously mentioned, individuals with gastric ulcers, gastritis, and other stomach disorders should limit their intake of any product containing aspirin. Even for those without stomach disorders, antacids containing aspirin are not recommended for upset stomach, for aspirin is the single most ingested gastric irritant. In fact, the most-often cited reasons for use of antacids (i.e., heartburn, upset stomach, and acid indigestion) represent situations in which aspirin should ave no place in the treatment. Also, alcohol and unbuffered aspirin exert a synergistic effect in promoting augmented blood loss from gastric mucosa.

The sodium contained in many antacids is another substance with possible side effects. Sodium promotes water retention and is contraindicated in those individuals with hypertension. Individuals on low-sodium diets should avoid sodium bicarbonate. Neither aluminum, magnesium, or calcium should be taken with the antibiotic Tetracycline, since they interfere with the absorption of this antibiotic from the gastrointestinal tract.

Antacids are usually safe and effective when taken as directed. However, the stomach empties rapidly and the neutralizing effect is lost within 30 minutes. If the condition persists, additional antacids must be consumed. Food, especially protein from lean meat or milk (skim milk is as good as whole), provides good natural neutralization of the gastric environment and produces less constipation than do antacids.

REGULATION OF NONPRESCRIPTION DRUGS

The fact that America is a chemical society can be understood in its fullest sense by viewing the thousands of advertisements and commercial messages that promote self-diagnosis by outlining symptoms. Although many suggest that one should see a doctor, they proclaim loudly that their product will do the job and at much less expense.

The public is also lulled into complacency by thinking that the legality of these substances ensures their effectiveness and safety. A brief look at the major legislative acts affecting over-the-counter drugs will indicate good intention, but a general lack of results. The first attempt at regulation came in 1906 with the passage of the Pure Food and Drug Act, which prohibited interstate commerce of adulterated or misbranded food and drugs. However, drugs did not have to be proven safe for human consumption until the passage of the Food, Drug, and Cosmetic Act of 1938. All *new* drugs coming onto the market had to be proven safe by the manufacturer and more carefully labeled. Still, old drugs did not come under the law and did not need to be proven safe. Also in 1938 the Wheeler-Lea amendment to the FTC Act provided additional control over false advertisement of drugs and cosmetics and over other deceptive practices not specified. In 1952 the Durham-Humphrey Amendment to the Food, Drug, and Cosmetic Act divided drugs into two classes: prescription and nonprescription. Finally, the Kefauver-Harris Amendment to the 1938 Food, Drug, and Cosmetic Act provided that the drug be proven not only safe, but effective. Again only new drugs came under the law's jurisdiction.

Thus, it would appear that the public is well protected; however, some problems still exist. For example, the National Academy of Sciences–National Research Council evaluated drugs introduced between 1938 and 1962 for effectiveness, and in relation to label claims, the panel concluded that only 15% of the drugs evaluated were effective. Twenty-seven percent were probably effective, but evidence was not

conclusive; 47% were possibly effective (again, the evidence presented was not con‐
clusive); and 11% were definitely ineffective. However, the major inadequacy o
this study was that only 400 of the estimated 100,000 to 500,000 OTC drugs wer
studied by this panel. The past decade has produced thousands of new drug prod‐
ucts, far too many for the Federal Food and Drug Administration to test. The gov
ernment has initiated a program of self-testing by pharmaceutical companies an
depends on their integrity for control. These companies, while basically honest
naturally "accentuate the positive and eliminate the negative." In recent senate hear‐
ings, testimony indicated that in case after case pharmaceutical companies have beer
guilty of misrepresenting, distorting, and even withholding information about thei
products. So a new approach has been initiated, centering on (1) the active in‐
gredients (it is estimated that only 200 different active ingredients make up the hun‐
dreds of thousands of OTC drugs), and (2) the intended purpose of the substance
Eventually 17 panels will review 26 categories of OTC drugs. The government wil
publish monographs specifying which ingredients may be included in products fo
treatment of a specified condition and will also specify the claims that may be mad
for that ingredient. Any manufacturer who exceeds the bounds of the monograph
would be required to file a New Drug Application with the FDA, proving both
safety and effectiveness of the drug.

New regulations concerning the deceptive advertising and labeling of OTC
drugs have also been adopted. Advertising is considered deceptive if an attempt is
made to conceal the active ingredient or if the manufacturer attempts to create new
markets by creating new diseases. A product is inadequately labeled (1) if all the
ingredients and amounts are not listed, (2) if the label makes exaggerated thera‐
peutic claims, (3) if warning statements are not prominent, and (4) if the warning
statements are not easily understood by lay people.

NONPRESCRIPTION DRUGS AS PART OF THE DRUG CULTURE

Over-the-counter medicines have been called ineffectual, innocuous, or mildly help‐
ful. While most authorities agree that if taken as directed they do little harm, it has
been pointed out that ineffectiveness often leads to overmedication and cross-
medication, and may be a legal path to drug misuse and abuse.

Indirectly, nonprescription drugs may contribute to an even more serious social
problem. The existence of so many drugs in the home, the ever-increasing reliance
on chemicals as cure-alls, and the massive amounts of advertising are suspected to
be related to the youthful drug scene of today. Advertising in general and drug
advertising in particular are seen as having a significant influence on illegal drug use.
The typical advertisement is composed of three parts: the first stage is the problem
or pain, the second stage brings on the pill, and the third stage is orgiastic ecstasy,
with everyone living happily ever after. The message of illegal drugs is in essence
the same as the OTC drugs: quick, easy escape or pleasure, immediate relief and

ratification, instant solution to all problems. The relationship between OTC drug
se and the use of illegal psychoactive drugs has been found in several studies. One
f the most publicized studies, conducted in New England, demonstrated an asso-
iation between (1) student use of popular OTC analgesics and the use of illegal
sychoactive agents, and (2) maternal use of OTC analgesics and the use of illegal
sychoactive agents by their children [4]. It may be that the same factors that con-
ribute to the overuse of OTC analgesics also permeate the use of illegal psychotropic
drugs, but it is even more likely that the students who use these drugs have developed a pattern of seeking a chemical resolution to their pain and problems. More
tudies of this nature are currently being conducted, but empirical evidence and
knowledge of the American drug scene would tend to make the results predictable.

REFERENCES

1. Beecher, H. K., "The Measurement of Pain," *Pharmacological Review,* 9:59–202, 1957.

2. Bernstein, S., and R. Leff, "Toxic Psychosis from Sleeping Medicine Containing Scopolamine," *New England Journal of Medicine,* 277:638–639, 1967.

3. Dipalma, J. R., ed., *Drills Pharmacology in Medicine.* New York: McGraw-Hill, 1971.

4. Estes, J. W., and M. Johnson, "Relationships among Medical and Nonmedical Uses of Pharmacologically Active Agents," *Clinical Pharmacology and Therapeutics,* 12(6):883–888, 1971.

5. Gleason, M. N., *et al., Clinical Toxicology of Commercial Products.* Baltimore: Williams and Wilkins, 1969.

6. Hollister, L. E., "Measuring Measurin: Problems of Oral Prolonged-Action Medications," *Clinical Pharmacology and Therapeutics,* 13(1):1–5, 1972.

7. Kales, J., *et al.,* "Are Over-the-Counter Sleep Medications Effective? All Night EEG Studies," *Current Therapeutic Research,* 13(3):143–151, 1971.

8. "Periodic Advice," *Moneysworth,* 2(11):2, 1972.

9. Rickels, K., "Drug, Doctor Warmth and Clinic Setting in the Symptomatic Response to Minor Tranquilizers," *Psychopharmacology,* 20:128–52, 1971.

10. Rickels, K., *et al.,* "Setting, Patient, and Doctor: Effects on Drug Response in Neurotic Patients," *Psychopharmacology,* 18:180–208, 1970.

11. Rickels, K., and P. Hesbacher, "OTC Daytime Sedatives," *Journal of the American Medical Association,* 223:29–33, 1973.

12. Shader, R. I., and D. J. Greenblatt, "Uses and Toxicity of Belladonna Alkaloids and Synthetic Anticholinergics," *Seminars in Psychiatry,* 3(4):449, 1971.

13. *The Democrat Chronicle,* Rochester, New York, Oct. 10, 1971.

14. Ullman, K. C., "Treatment of Scopolamine-Induced Delirium," *Lancet,* January 31, 1970.

SUGGESTED READING

Armstrong, J. B., "Overmedicated Society," *Canadian Medical Association Journal* 112(4):413, 1975.

Babb, R. R., "Constipation and Laxative Abuse," *Western Journal of Medicine*, 122(1) 93–96, 1975.

Bell, S. A., *et al.*, "Drug Blood Levels as Indices in Evaluation of a Sustained-Release Aspirin," *Journal of New Drugs*, 6:284–304, 1966.

Cummings, J. H., "Laxative Abuse," *Gut*, 15(9):758–766, 1974.

"Dangers from 'Over the Counter' Drugs," *Medical News-Tribune*, 4:3, 1972.

"FDA Begins Inventory of All Drugs Currently Marketed for Human Use," *FDA Papers*, 5:33, 1971.

Griffenhager, G. B., ed., *Handbook of Nonprescription Drugs.* Washington, D.C.: American Pharmaceutical Association, 1969.

Hasebroock, W. H., "Home Remedies in Household Management," *Academy of Sciences* 120(2):1005, 1965.

Hobson, A. J., "Sleep after Exercise," *Science*, 162:1503–1505, 1968.

Kales, A., and J. D. Kales, "Sleep Laboratory and Evaluation of Psychoactive Drugs,' *Pharmacology for Physicians*, 4:1–6, 1970.

Leff, R., and S. Bernstein, "Proprietary Hallucinogens," *Diseases of the Nervous System*, 29:621, 1968.

Modell, W., ed., *Drugs of Choice 1970–1971.* St. Louis: C. V. Mosby, 1970.

Muller, D. J., "Unpublicized Hallucinogens: the Dangerous Belladonna Alkaloids," *Journal of the American Medical Association*, 202:650, 1967.

Parkhouse, J., *et al.*, "The Clinical Dose Response to Aspirin," *British Journal of Anaesthesiology*, 40:440, 1968.

Purnell, J., and A. F. Burry, "Analgesic Consumption in a Country Town," *Journal of Clinical Pharmacology*, 7:10, 1967.

Rickels, K., ed., *Nonspecific Factors in Drug Therapy.* Springfield, Ill.: Charles C. Thomas, 1968.

Silverman, M. M., and P. R. Lee, *Pills, Profits and Politics.* Berkeley: University of California Press, 1974.

Stroo, H. H., "A Case of Transient Schizophrenia Due to Scopolamine Poisoning," *Virginia Medical Monthly*, 94:107, 1967.

Tempero, K. F., and D. B. Hunninghake, "Antihistamines," *Postgraduate Medicine*, 48:149, 1970.

"When Relief of Pain is the Challenge: Selecting the Right Analgesic for Your Patient," *Patient Care*, 6:22–53, 1972.

Wood, C. D., and A. Graybiel, "A Theory of Motion Sickness Based on Pharmacological Reactions," *Clinical Pharmacology and Therapeutics*, 11:621, 1970.

11 DRUGS AND THE LAW

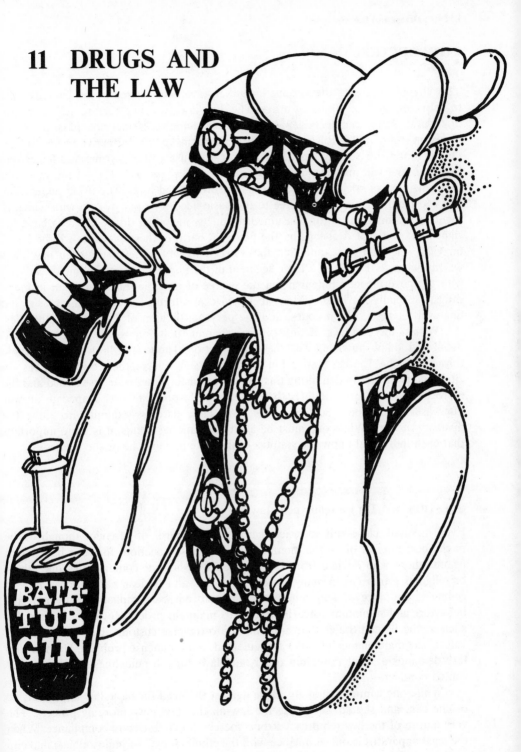

INTRODUCTION

This chapter discusses the various laws that have been passed in the United States to help cope with the abuse of drugs. The drug laws now in force are a combination of federal, state, and local laws that have accumulated since the passage of the Harrison Act of 1914. Restriction of drug use seems to arise from two basic motives. One is moral, for society has deemed most drug use morally wrong and hopes that the drug laws will protect the user from his own "weakness." The second motive is the protection of society from potential harm inflicted by a drug-using population.

Most individuals would agree to the basic need for some system with which to regulate the distribution of consumed products, including drugs. Citizens have the right to expect that decisions on the potential harm of these products will be based on valid scientific facts, and that these decisions will be reversed when new facts warrant change. Recently, a large segment of the population has become dissatisfied with the government's judgment on the degree of potential harm inherent in many drugs, especially marijuana. Many feel that legal reforms are at the mercy of vested financial interests, moral codes, and the personal opinion of legislative authorities.

Within the confines of one general chapter, it is impossible to cover in full detail all the laws involved with the drug question. The federal laws are enforceable throughout the United States, but individual states have their own laws, as do cities and counties. In delimiting this vast area, existing laws were researched and the more pertinent information (both legal and philosophical) was shaped to answer often-asked questions. Several states have been used as examples to show the diversity of laws. While one must be aware of national trends, it is more important that each individual know the statutes of the state in which he or she resides.

QUESTION 1:   Do we really need laws?

Even in small, close-knit societies there exist standards of behavior thought to be in the best interest of all the members, and negative sanctions that can be brought against those who deviate from these standards. Societies comprised of one ethnic or religious group (as in many European, Asian, and African nations) can rely on general acceptance of longstanding tradition to ensure compliance with expected behavior, and minimum force is needed to maintain order. However, in societies such as the United States that are made up of diverse customs, beliefs, and moral values, the maintenance of order has emerged as an immense problem. Human welfare demands at least minimum order, and laws furnish guidelines for socially accepted conduct.

While one cannot rationally argue against the need for basic law and order, he or she can, and should, scrutinize the law-making and law-enforcing process. The very nature of the law requires a strong coercive force to ensure compliance. When the legal apparatus is out of balance with the ethnic, social, or philosophical makeup of the people, equality is hard to maintain.

If order and socially accepted conduct can be maintained only by the negative threats of the legal establishment, a police state will surely evolve. Laws must be but a baseline of human protection, with most actual social interaction being conducted on a much higher ethical level. It is indeed odd that many businessmen regard as ethical practice anything that laws have not been passed against, while at the same time expecting a high ethical code from the religious, educational, and professional institutions that serve them. Such double standards and inequalities not only make laws necessary, but also promote the growth of a much larger, more stringent legal system than would otherwise be necessary [9].

QUESTION 2: Does strict regulation of social conduct encourage contempt for the law?

The answer to this question would probably be "yes." Many of our laws are merely statements of moral code, and exist to satisfy the conscience of society by condemning acts that are thought to be immoral. If the laws that make a criminal offense of some kinds of sexual behavior between married adults, of illnesses such as alcoholism and drug addiction, and of oral obscenity and disorderly conduct were strictly enforced, half of the adult population of our country would be behind bars! These laws remain unrepealed, so as not to give the impression of moral decay; enforcement is inconsistent and dependent on the philosophy of the law enforcement officer and on the offender. In recent years, "hippies" or teenagers who appear with current hair and clothing fashions have been seen as undesirables, and have borne the wrath of social and legal prejudice.

Laws enforced against conduct that is deemed normal by large segments of the population do breed contempt for the system. Recently, young adults throughout the country were urged to appear en masse at their local police station bearing a marijuana joint in hand to force arrests for possession. It is apparent that much of the contemporary disobedience to law is as much an attempt to harass authorities into concessions to legal reform as it is an attempt to practice individual liberties. For the legal system, or for that matter the whole society, to survive, it must be able to accommodate dissent. It has been said many times that, in a democracy, dissent is the first step toward progress.

In recent years much has been written about the right to violate unjust laws. This idea is not new; it was seen in the writings of Plato and, technically, was written into our Declaration of Independence. Justification for this right evolves from the existence of a higher "natural law" from which human laws should be derived. Martin Luther King wrote that a just law is a "man-made law of God" and an unjust law is a code that is "out of harmony with moral law" [9].

Two important questions, then, must be considered. Can order be maintained when large segments of the population are frustrated by the rule of laws they feel are unjust? And can our democracy survive with a legal establishment that is not responsive to the needs and wishes of the people?

The contract between the government and the governed (the Constitution) does have some built-in provisions protecting dissent. Freedom of speech, political rights,

voting rights, freedom to assemble, and freedom to petition the government are bu
a few. Individuals or groups are free to use any of these to convince officials of th
need for changes [11].

All too often it is not the law that erodes basic rights, but the fears and preju
dices of the people. The result of legal dissent or nonconformity often is loss o
employment or expulsion from school. Society must be convinced that frustration
engendered by denial of basic rights are the beginning of the end of our democracy

QUESTION 3:   Do drug laws cause overcriminalization in our society?

It is common knowledge that the law enforcement structure is having difficulty keep
ing pace with the rising incidence of crime. One often cited reason is the drain or
law enforcement resources caused by overconcern with criminal prosecution o
"crimes without victims." Crimes without victims are activities that large segment
of the population consider normal. They are "crimes" committed between consent-
ing adults or "crimes" in which the defendants are the victims, such as narcotic
addiction *per se*.

The costs of this overconcern for crimes without victims are (a) a drain of man-
power away from the fight against more serious crimes of violence, (b) demoraliza-
tion of police officers who must act as undercover agents to buy drugs or make
advances to homosexuals and prostitutes, (c) attraction of organized crime, which
is willing to take higher risks for higher profits and therefore constantly increases the
prices of drugs, and (d) most important, frustration and contempt for a legal system that punishes crimes of illness or involuntary action, like most alcoholism and
drug addiction [10].

Recent sociological conditions, such as the use of drugs in the youth subculture,
have increased the incidence of drug use to the point where 30 million have experimented with marijuana and countless others are using psychedelics, stimulants,
and depressants. These facts necessitate new attitudes toward drug users. Sanctions
against drug dependence must be continued, but legal penalties must yield to medical treatment as initially outlined in the Narcotic Addict Rehabilitation Act of 1966.

Laws against the possession of marijuana must be reevaluated in light of the
current evidence indicating that marijuana is not addictive and has little long-range
physical effect. There appears to be little justification for the felony convictions
imposed on marijuana users [10].

QUESTION 4:   Are drug laws going to stop the abuse of drugs? If not, why have
them?

The answer to this question depends on whether you view the laws as a total deterrent to drug use or as a helper in an effort by the whole society. The obvious fact is
that law enforcement used alone has been a failure. Drug abuse has steadily increased despite stronger laws and increasingly severe penalties. Many proponents of
drug use have indicated that the law itself is the most harmful aspect of marijuana
use. To be sure, many individuals have been deterred from drug use out of fear of
legal punishment. But all too often the chronic drug user with emotional difficulties

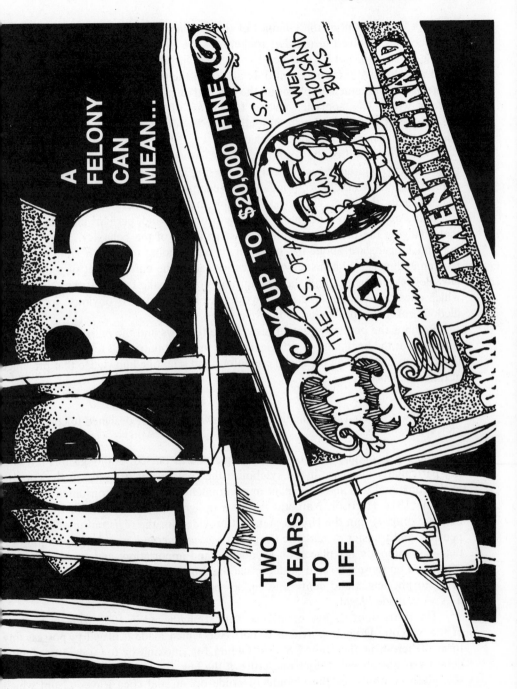

does not operate within the confines of the established mores or laws. The person who becomes involved in murder, robbery, or the use of drugs is usually convinced that he or she will not be detected by the legal authorities.

Laws do have their part, but only a part, in the total effort of society to protect its members. Too much emphasis on the law and on punishment has not worked, and will not work. This approach gives a false sense of security to those who see it as the answer to a problem which, in reality, can be solved only by effective education and resultant changes in societal behavior.

When the mood of the country changes, law will also change. When there is a public outcry, legislators act quickly by passing new laws. As the perceived threat diminishes, one would expect the law to be changed to reflect that attitude, but such is not usually the case. The reasons for this may be that as public interest wanes legislators move on to other more pressing problems, and, perhaps more important, that changing the law would indicate a sanctioning of the behavior. While society may no longer care about the behavior, it is not going to give the impression of recommending it. What usually changes instead is the enforcement of a particular law. Police and district and states' attorneys do not make laws, but they do choose which ones they will enforce most vigorously. The problem is obvious: some jurisdictions enforce a particular code while others do not.

Perhaps the best way to gain insight into the laws and the reasons behind them is to start at the beginning of drug legislation in our country and follow it through to the present, highlighting the social conditions and scientific knowledge that prevailed at different times.

QUESTION 5:   What were the first federal laws specifically designed to control drug abuse?

In 1906 the Federal Pure Food and Drug Act was passed. Although this law was not particularly effective, it did symbolize the concern for drug use in the country at that time and was an experiment in government control over consumed products.

The 1914 Harrison Narcotic Act was designed to control the distribution of narcotic drugs within the United States. It provided for the registration of sales, dispensing, and transfer of narcotic drugs. Its *modus operandi* was the imposition of a tax—a commodity tax placed on production and importation, and an occupational tax placed on those who sold or dispensed the drug. By restricting the use of narcotic drugs to physicians and dentists in cases where it was medically advised, all other uses were made illegal.

The restrictions against opiate use were strengthened in 1922 with the passage of the Narcotic Drug Import and Export Act, which made it illegal to possess any form of heroin in the United States. Opium for smoking or for use in producing heroin was also illegal. Under the terms of the law, the Commissioner of Narcotics was given control over the amount of crude opium and coca leaves (from which cocaine is derived) which would be needed to supply medical and scientific needs [6].

QUESTION 6: What were the prevailing attitudes and the available information leading to the passage of these acts?

The stimulus for passage of the two latter laws—the Harrison Narcotic Act and the Narcotic Drug Import and Export Act—came from evidence that an ever-increasing number of persons were becoming addicted to opium and its derivatives. There was a growing awareness that many legal patent medicines contained narcotics. (Indeed, some of these patent medicines containing morphine were advertised as cures for opium addiction!) Still fresh in the minds of legislators of that day were stories of Civil War casualties becoming addicted to morphine, Chinese opium smoking, and the realization that narcotic drugs could be purchased or diverted from pharmacies and wholesalers with relative ease.

QUESTION 7: Was the early prohibition of drugs directed toward other depressants, stimulants, and the psychedelics?

The early drugs covered under the Harrison Act were classified as "habit-forming narcotic drugs" and consisted of opium and its derivatives, heroin and morphine, and coca leaves and their principal derivative, cocaine.

The federal government did not then and does not now attempt to classify drugs in a medical sense (as psychedelics, depressants, etc.). It regulates a drug only because it is believed to be dangerous and/or habit-forming.

QUESTION 8: When was marijuana first brought under legal control of the federal government?

In 1937 the Marijuana Tax Act was passed. Like the early opium laws, this was part of the Code of the Internal Revenue Department, but was clearly an attempt to apply federal police powers to marijuana regulation and enforcement.

This act provided that a tax be paid by all persons who imported, manufactured, produced, compounded, sold, dealt in, dispensed, prescribed, administered, or gave away marijuana. The tax for those registered under the act was one dollar per ounce; for those not registered it was a hundred dollars per ounce [8].

QUESTION 9: Have penalties under the Marijuana Tax Act increased or decreased since its passage?

The original maximum penalty was a $2000 fine and/or five years in prison, and probation or suspended sentence was possible. Working from the basic belief that the answer to the problem of drug use, and of other crimes as well, was increased penalties, the government gradually increased them. However, portions of this act were voided as unconstitutional as a result of the *Timothy F. Leary* vs. *United States* decision of 1969 in which the act of declaring possession in order to pay the required marijuana tax was ruled to be self-incriminating.

In 1951 the Boggs Act outlined the penalties, as shown in the following table, for anyone violating the federal narcotics laws.

	Fine		Imprisonment
First offense*	$1000 to $2000	and	2 to 5 years
Second offense	$1000 to $2000	and	5 to 10 years
Third offense	$1000 to $2000	and	10 to 20 years

* First offenders can receive probation or suspended sentence.

In 1956 penalties were again increased in the Narcotics Control Act, and agai in 1960 in the Narcotics Manufacturing Act. Separate penalties were established fo possession and sale of narcotics or marijuana [2]:

	Fine		Imprisonment*
Possession			
First offense	up to $20,000	and	2 to 10 years
Second offense	up to $20,000	and	5 years to life
Third offense	up to $20,000	and	10 years to life
Sale to adult			
First offense	up to $20,000	and	5 to 20 years
Second offense	up to $20,000	and	10 years to life
Third offense	up to $20,000	and	10 years to life

* No probation or suspension of sentence allowed.

The first major medical and rehabilitative legislation emerged with the passage of the Narcotic Addict Rehabilitation Act of 1966. It provided for (a) civil commitment of certain addicts in lieu of prosecution for federal offenses, (b) sentencing of addicts to commitment for treatment after conviction of federal offenses, (c) civil commitment of persons not charged with a criminal offense, (d) rehabilitation and post-hospitalization cure programs, and assistance to states and localities, and (e) availability of parole to all marijuana violators currently incarcerated or subsequently convicted under federal law.

As the drug problem crept quietly into the white middle class, the mood of the country continued to change. In 1970 concerned legislators, prodded by an impressive contingent of educators, researchers, and rehabilitation personnel, passed the most comprehensive drug control act in our history, aptly named the Comprehensive Drug Abuse Prevention and Control Act. With significant amendments made on July 1, 1971, this act replaced the more than 50 separate laws previously enacted.

This law, as amended, accomplished the following:

1. Enforcement authority was taken out of the hands of the Treasury Department and given to the Bureau of Narcotics and Dangerous Drugs (BNDD). This direct control of drugs replaced the confusing attempts at control through excise taxes. Subsequently the new Drug Enforcement Administration (DEA) was created to uniformly enforce drug laws.

2. It simplified the classification problem by creating five categories (schedules) ased not on chemical nature but on the potential for abuse and the need or medical se of the substance.

Schedule I contains those substances that have no recognized medical use and have high potential for abuse. Some popular examples are heroin, marijuana, peyote, mescaline, LSD, DET, DMT, and THC (see Glossary for chemical names). Prescription provisions do not apply to these drugs because their only legal use is for research, not for the practice of medicine.

Schedule II is made up of those drugs formerly known as "class A narcotics" plus he amphetamines. These drugs have some medical use, but possess a high potential or abuse. Some examples are codeine, opium, morphine, Dilaudid, Dolophine Methadone), Demerol, Benzedrine, Dexedrine, Dexamyl, Bamadex, Ambar, Methedrine, Desoxyn, and cocaine. More recently included in this group as drugs of high buse potential are amobarbital, pentobarbital, secobarbital, methaqualone, and Tuinal. In order to obtain these drugs, a written prescription is required, and this prescription cannot be refilled, as can prescriptions for Schedule III, IV, or V drugs.

Schedule III is made up of drugs formerly known as "class B narcotics," as well as ome nonnarcotic depressants and some nonamphetamine stimulants. These drugs ave a moderate to high potential for abuse and are used medically. Some popular xamples are paregoric, Emperin with codeine, ASA with codeine, Doriden, Preudin, and Ritalin. A prescription is needed and may be refilled up to five times in ix months.

Schedule IV contains drugs that have low potential for abuse and are used in medicine. Some examples are phenobarbital, chloral hydrate, paraldehyde, Equanil, and Miltown. A prescription is needed and may be refilled up to five times in six months.

Schedule V contains drugs formerly known as "exempt narcotics" such as cough yrups containing codeine. Prescription requirements are the same as those for Schedules III and IV.

3. It established more stringent penalties for pushers, dealers, and those involved n organized crime, and placed lesser penalties on the user (compare the penalties under the Boggs Act and Narcotics Manufacturing Act previously mentioned).

	Fine		Imprisonment
Possession			
First offense	up to $ 5,000	and	1 year*
Second offense	up to $10,000	and	2 years
Sale			
First offense	up to $25,000	and	15 years
Second offense	up to $50,000	and	30 years

* Probation or suspension allowed.

4. It provided for liberal appropriations of funds for research and education.

5. It provided for appropriations for several hundred more agents to aid in enforce ment of the act.

6. It established a commission to study marijuana (see Question 11).

It remains difficult to list specific laws and penalties for each state because of th variance that exists. Many states are in the process of making long-overdue change in their statutes. The present system allows for too much inequality by allowing to great a difference between states and too wide a range of penalties. The feder statutes serve as guidelines for the states. The reader is urged to research state an local statutes, for it is the local laws that will apply to the offender.

QUESTION 10:   Considering what we know about marijuana, why is the law again its use so harsh?

It appears to be easier to make laws than to change them. The Marijuana Tax Ac (1937) and Uniform Narcotic Drug Act (1932) are both quite old, and one mus consider the information that was available when the lawmakers formed their opin ions concerning marijuana.

First, one must consider that marijuana did not command all the publicity does today, nor did it enjoy such widespread use. In the 1930s it was used primaril by ghetto dwellers, jazz musicians, people of the "night life"—a small, easily over looked, minority segment of society. Since these people were far removed from th mainstream of life and were causing no problem, there was little advertisement o marijuana use. Because of the low positions that marijuana smokers held in society it was easy for the "public" to look down on them, condemn their actions, and pas laws to "help" them. There was little scientific investigation into the physiological psychological, or social harm of marijuana. Consequently, the information receive by the public came mainly from empirical observations of law enforcement person nel who dealt with problem cases. Since marijuana was so strongly associated wit heroin, the marijuana user was assumed to have the same characteristics as th heroin addict. Marijuana was accused of being the cause of violent crimes, including murder and rape. The crime reports and newspapers told of individuals who as saulted children and peace officers while under the influence of marijuana, and gav detailed reports of body dismemberment and other insane acts purportedly cause by users of marijuana.

Congressional hearings were conducted, and evidence of alleged mental and physical deterioration resulting from marijuana use combined with a massive anti marijuana campaign put on by the Federal Bureau of Narcotics convinced Congress that it had no choice but to rule that marijuana was a harmful, addicting drug like heroin and that it should be controlled in a similar manner.

The only spokesman against the proposed marijuana laws at the congressional hearings was a representative of a birdseed manufacturer. However, shortly afterward, Mayor Fiorello LaGuardia of New York ordered the New York Academy of Medicine to study the problem. After years of study they concluded that there was no evidence to link marijuana with crime (the major focus of the arguments of Harry Anslinger, then director of the Bureau of Narcotics), and that there was little conclusive evidence that marijuana was harmful to health. Some years later the assertion that marijuana caused criminal behavior was dropped, but that made little difference—penalties continued to increase with the passage of subsequent laws.

QUESTION 11: In light of the increased knowledge of marijuana, has the law changed?

Few changes have been made despite increased scientific information and reports, such as the White House Conference on Narcotic and Drug Abuse, which indicated that the dangers of marijuana use have been exaggerated and that long-term prison sentences for occasional users and possessors are not in the best interest of society [8]. Similar findings with more documentation and authority have been reported by the Commission on Marijuana and Drug Abuse. This commission, chaired by former Pennsylvania governor Raymond Shafer, was part of the Comprehensive Drug Abuse Prevention and Control Act of 1970. The committee submitted extensive reports to the President and Congress early in 1972. While the report fell short of recommending that marijuana be legalized, it suggested that the penalty for private use be lessened to a misdemeanor or abolished altogether. Although the likelihood of imprisonment (especially for the first offense) for possession is decreasing, no uniform code is followed.

QUESTION 12: What are the laws and penalties for the use of barbiturates, amphetamines, and substances like LSD?

Although the use of these substances was not a major problem in 1938, the Federal Food, Drug, and Cosmetic Act was passed in this year to control prescription as well as over-the-counter (OTC) drugs. This act drew attention to misuse and abuse of drugs that were basically safe when used as prescribed. Subsequent amendments of this act provided stronger regulations against the manufacture, distribution, and possession of prescribed drugs, in addition to setting up penalties for illegal traffic in them.

The Durham-Humphrey Amendment of 1951 provided even stronger control of prescribed barbiturates and amphetamines. Other amendments since that time have classified synthetic hallucinogens such as LSD as dangerous drugs and set up strong penalties for their possession and sale [5].

Penalties for illegal possession of dangerous drugs vary from state to state. Some states have passed new laws to deal with them, while others have modified existing laws. The Drug Abuse Control Amendments to the Federal Food, Drug, and Cosmetic Act, which were passed in 1965 and amended in 1968, set down the following provisions [3].

	Fine		Imprisonment
Possession			
First offense	$1 to $1000	or	1 year maximum
Second offense	$1 to $1000	or	1 year maximum
Third offense	$1 to $1000	or	3 years maximum
Sale			
First offense	$1 to $15,000	and/or	5 years maximum
Second offense	$1 to $20,000	and/or	10 years maximum

* If the conditions of parole are met, conviction can be set aside.
† Parole allowed, but no reversal of conviction.

The formerly classified Dangerous Drugs are now controlled by the Comprehen
sive Drug Abuse Prevention and Control Act of 1970. In this act the hallucinogen:
are placed in Schedule I, and amphetamines and most barbiturates in Schedule I
(see Question 9).

Again, penalties vary from state to state. However, in most states possession o
unprescribed pep pills or depressants is a misdemeanor. In 1968 California passed ε
law allowing the judge to give a misdemeanor sentence (one year or less in a county
jail) or a felony sentence (one to ten years in a state prison) for first-offens
possession of either marijuana or a restricted dangerous drug [1].

Many states provide for closer control over prescribed drugs by demanding tha
all prescriptions be filled out in triplicate, one copy being kept by the physician, one
by the pharmacist, and the third being sent to the Bureau of Narcotic Enforcement

While the statutes usually classify possession of dangerous drugs as a misde
meanor, with a $1 to $3000 fine and a prison term of up to one year, conviction for
sale can bring from 10 years to life imprisonment.

QUESTION 13:   Do the restrictions on the use of hallucinogens violate one's freedom of religion?

Several cases concerning the use of psychedelics have been tested on the grounds of
religious freedom. The cases of *California* vs. *Woody* in 1969, *United States* vs.
Leary in 1967, and *United States* vs. *Kuch* in 1968 are a few examples. In the first
of these the Supreme Court of California held that the use of peyote was a corner-
stone of the religion in question and that its use was protected by the Constitution.
However, in most states, members of the Native American Church (the religion in
question in this case) must be of one-quarter Indian blood and be registered by the
state, and all peyote used must be secured from legal sources and registered.

In both the Leary and Kuch cases the courts rejected the argument that the
Constitution protected the use of hallucinogenic substances. They concluded that
the use of hallucinogens constituted a threat to society and that overt acts prompted
by religious belief are not totally free from legislative restrictions. Although the
Native American Church has been able to prove that peyote is essential to its religious practice, neither the Neo-American (in the Leary case) nor the Hindu religion (in the Kuch case) has been able to establish this foundation [4].

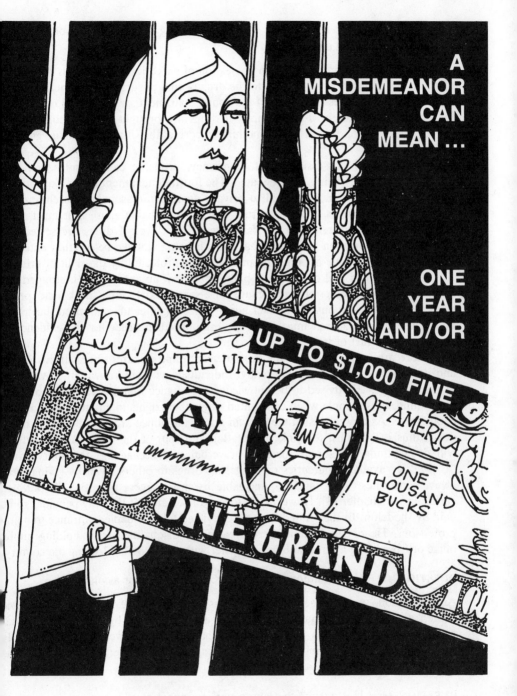

QUESTION 14:   Must the narcotic or dangerous drug be on one's person before h or she can be accused of possession?

A person may be presumed to be in possession of narcotics or dangerous drugs if h or she is found to be close enough to the drug or in a position to manipulate or us the drug. In most cases the owner of the house, apartment, or car is held responsibl for drugs found therein. For example, if drugs are brought to your house by ai invited guest at a party and you do nothing to correct the situation, you are guilty c possession.

The issues of possession, right to privacy, probable cause, and search ani seizure are currently being hotly debated. The fourth amendment to the Constitutioi protects the right of an individual to privacy against unreasonable search and sei zures. Authorities must have a warrant based on probable cause that must stani up in court as being real and not fabricated. Thus, even if drugs are seized, thi police must have reason to believe that a law is being violated before they enter thi premises. However, the act must be private to be protected by the right of privacy If a door is opened and drugs are in plain sight, or if an automobile is stopped ani drugs are plainly visible, probable cause for a search exists. The "no knock" provi sions under the Omnibus Crime Act allow police to enter unannounced, but prob able cause for the search must be firmly established in order for the evidence ti stand up in a court of law.

There are no absolutes in the area of search and seizure, since various judge: and juries will see situations differently. Individuals who are knowingly in violatioi of the law are well advised to be knowledgeable of such matters. Unbelievable as i may sound, most people when confronted waive their rights in an attempt to appeai cooperative. As any television viewer can attest, the police are not allowed to maki deals; thus it is foolish to think cooperation and spur-of-the-moment explanation: will do anything but supply material or verbal evidence against the guilty party

Making available narcotics or dangerous drugs to others, even by giving them away, constitutes "sale" and is punishable by more severe penalties, as outlinec earlier in the chapter [3]. However, prison and fines are not the only penalties to be paid by the felon. In the United States a convicted felon is denied entrance to many professions. He or she cannot carry firearms, is disqualified from holding public office or from being a juror, and must register with police before leaving the country.

QUESTION 15:   Can an automobile be searched for drugs or alcohol?

An automobile may be searched for drugs or intoxicating liquor on "probable cause," that is, on reasonable grounds of belief supported by circumstances that would warrant a cautious man to believe that such items were being unlawfully transported in that automobile. In many states, the automobile must be forfeited as penalty if liquor or drugs are found [12].

QUESTION 16:   Is it against the law to possess model glue?

Many states have passed laws against the possession of model glue by persons under the age of 21. Many cities have ordinances against the possession of model glue,

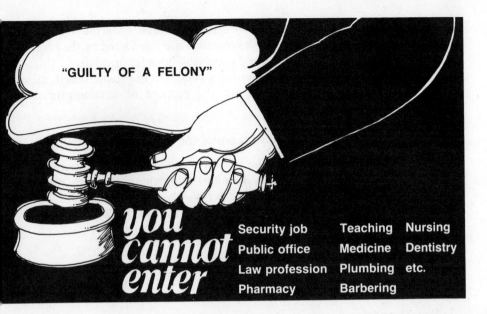

"GUILTY OF A FELONY"

you cannot enter

Security job	Teaching	Nursing
Public office	Medicine	Dentistry
Law profession	Plumbing	etc.
Pharmacy	Barbering	

adhesive cement, or plastic solvent which contains toluene, acetone, xylene, butyl alcohol, hexane, tricresyl phosphate, or other toxic ingredients. This offense is considered a misdemeanor punishable by 90 days in jail, but some cities have penalties of up to $200 and/or a jail sentence of up to six months.

The primary problem is that in most cases the offender is a juvenile. It is very difficult to punish the salesperson, for he or she does not know the intent of the buyer. In cities with ordinances against model glue, a juvenile must have the written consent of his or her parent or guardian in order to purchase this substance [7].

QUESTION 17: If a person is found to be addicted to a drug but not in possession of drugs, what, if anything, can the laws do?

In most states it is unlawful for a person to be addicted to the use of narcotic drugs, including barbituric acid and its derivatives (barbiturates). Although this is a misdemeanor punishable by a 90-day jail sentence, the addict, by physician's certificate and at the discretion of the court, is usually committed to a correctional institution or hospital for treatment. The time of release from the hospital is determined by the head of the institution, who certifies that the person has been sufficiently treated.

QUESTION 18: What is the penalty for possession of alcohol by a minor?

The illegal possession of alcohol by a minor (a person under 21 in most states) is a misdemeanor and usually punishable by a $10 to $100 fine. It is important to note the term "illegal possession," for not all possession is illegal for a minor.

QUESTION 19: What is the penalty for the sale of intoxicating liquor to a minor?

As is the case with all legislation concerning intoxicating liquor, the statutes vary greatly from state to state, but to be guilty, the seller must know that the minor is i fact a minor. Appearance and body development are considered by the court to de termine whether or not the minor could reasonably pass for an adult.

In most states it is a misdemeanor for a person to use fraud, deceit, misrepre sentation, or a false name or facts for the purpose of obtaining intoxicatin liquor [12].

QUESTION 20:   What is the penalty for possession of cigarettes by a minor?

Although it is technically against the law for a minor (under 16 years of age o under 18 years of age, depending on the state) to purchase cigarettes, there is usu ally no fine for this offense. However, the person who sells the cigarettes is guilty c a misdemeanor and is usually fined between $10 and $100 [12].

REFERENCES

1. *California Health and Safety Code.* Sacramento, 1965.

2. Fact Sheet from Bureau of Narcotics and Dangerous Drugs, U.S. Department o Justice. Washington, D.C., 1969.

3. Fact Sheet: Drug Abuse Control Amendments of 1965, Food and Drug Administra tion, U.S. Department of Health, Education, and Welfare. Washington, D.C., 1969

4. *Handbook of Federal Narcotic and Dangerous Drug Laws,* pp. 72–73. Washington D.C.: Bureau of Narcotics and Dangerous Drugs, 1969.

5. Jones, K. L., *et al., Drugs, Alcohol and Tobacco.* San Francisco: Harper and Row 1970.

6. Kaplan, R., *Drug Abuse: Perspective on Drugs.* Dubuque, Ia.: William C. Brown 1970.

7. Kupperstein, L. R., and R. M. Susman, "A Bibliography on the Inhalation of Glue Fumes and Other Toxic Vapors," *International Journal of Addictions,* 3:177–197 1968.

8. *Proceedings: White House Conference on Narcotic and Drug Abuse.* Washington, D.C., September, 1963.

9. Report of the National Commission on the Causes and Prevention of Violence, "Civil Disobedience," in *To Establish Justice and to Insure Domestic Tranquility,* pp. 87–118. Washington, D.C.: U.S. Government Printing Office, 1969.

10. Report of the National Commission on the Causes and Prevention of Violence, "The Problem of Over-Criminalization," in *Law and Order Reconsidered,* pp. 551–567. Washington, D.C.: U.S. Government Printing Office, 1969.

11. Report of the National Commission on the Causes and Prevention of Violence, "Violence and Law Enforcement," in *To Establish Justice and to Insure Domestic Tranquility,* pp. 139–167. Washington, D.C.: U.S. Government Printing Office, 1969.

12. *Vernon's Penal Code of the State of Texas.* Kansas City, Mo.: Vernon's Law Book Company, 1970.

SUGGESTED READING

Adams, Thomas F., *Law Enforcement: an Introduction to the Police Role in the Community.* Englewood Cliffs, N.J.: Prentice-Hall, 1968.

Buse, Renée, *The Deadly Silence.* New York: Doubleday, 1965.

California Alcoholic Beverage Control Department, *Questions and Answers Concerning the Alcoholic Beverage Control Act and Related Constitutional Provisions.* Sacramento, 1965.

California, *Delinquency Prevention Commission, Drugs.* Sacramento, 1964.

California Youth Authority, *An Exploratory Study of the Narcotic Control Program for Youth Authority Parolees (a Preliminary Report),* by George F. Davis. Sacramento, 1964.

Conigan, Robert L., *Chemical Tests and the Law: Legal Aspects of the Constitutional Issues Involved in Chemical Tests to Determine Alcoholic Influence.* Evanston, Ill.: Traffic Institute, Northwestern University, 1957.

deFaubert Maunder, M. J., "The Rapid Detection of Drugs of Addiction," *Medicine, Science and Law,* 14(4):243–249, 1974.

Del Piombo, Akbar, *Fuzz Against Junk: the Saga of the Narcotics Brigade.* New York: Citadel, 1960.

Eldridge, William B., *Narcotics and the Law: a Critique of the American Experiment in Narcotic Drug Control,* 2nd ed. Chicago: University of Chicago Press, 1967.

Gaffney, G. H., "The Position of the Bureau of Narcotics," *Illinois Medical Journal,* 130:516–520, 1966.

Gale, W. C., "Why Not Legalize Narcotics?" San Diego: Publisher's Export, 1967.

Harney, Malachi L., and J. C. Cross, *Narcotic Officer's Notebook.* Springfield, Ill.: Charles C. Thomas, 1961.

Hess, C., "New Trends in Narcotic Addiction Control," *Public Health Report,* 81:277–281, 1966.

Inciardi, J. A., and C. D. Chambers, eds., *Drugs and the Criminal Justice System.* Beverly Hills, Calif.: Sage, 1974.

"Information for Law Enforcement Agencies." Washington, D.C.: Bureau of Drug Abuse Control, Federal Drug Administration, July 21, 1966.

Kiev, Ari, *The Drug Epidemic.* New York: Free Press, 1975.

Lindesmith, A. R., *The Addict and the Law.* Bloomington: Indiana University Press, 1965.

Moscow, Alvin, *Merchants of Heroin; In-Depth Portrayal of Business in the Underworld.* New York: Dial, 1968.

Murton, T., ed., *Law Enforcement and Dangerous Drug Abuse.* Berkeley: University of California Press, 1966.

Siragusa, Charles, *The Trail of the Poppy (Behind the Mask of the Mafia).* Englewood Cliffs, N.J.: Prentice-Hall, 1966.

United States Commission on Narcotic Drugs, *Narcotic Drugs under International Control.* Geneva: United Nations, 1963.

United States Narcotics Bureau, *Prescribing and Dispensing of Narcotics Under Harrison Narcotic Law*. Washington, D.C.: U.S. Government Printing Office, 1966.

United States President's Commission on Law Enforcement and the Administration of Justice, *Narcotics and Drug Abuse*. Washington, D.C.: U.S. Government Printing Office, 1967.

United States Task Force on Narcotics and Drug Abuse, *Task Force Report: Narcotics and Drug Abuse*. Washington, D.C.: U.S. Government Printing Office, 1967.

LAW-RELATED TERMINOLOGY

Big John	The police
Bust	Drug raid
Fuzz	The police
Heat	Police investigation
Man	The police
Narc	Narcotics officer
Sam	Narcotics agent of the federal government
Uncle	Federal officer

12 ON BEING HIGH

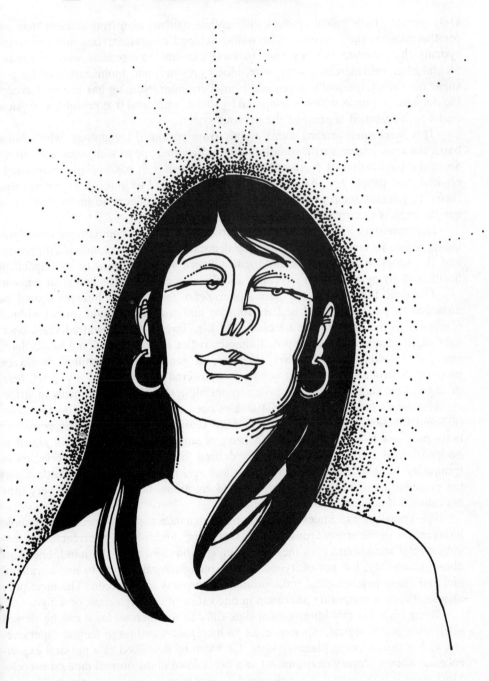

INTRODUCTION

Only minute physiological changes differentiate modern man from ancient man or for that matter, the caveman. The well-developed central nervous and endocrine systems that allowed the caveman to meet physical emergencies with increasing mental alertness, increased heart rate, blood pressure, and mobilization of fat and sugar for energy is equally developed in modern man. Nothing has changed except the outward response, which is tempered by social conditions that prohibit a physical outlet to heightened arousal of the nervous system.

This heightened arousal stems mainly from advanced technology, which bombards the consciousness with stimuli that must be either coped with or escaped from. Since the publication of Norbert Wiener's *Cybernetics,* it has become increasingly obvious that people are so dependent on machines and technology in general that their life pursuits seem to be an endless technological education in an attempt to use the tireless electrical helpers more efficiently.

Industrialization, forced urban development with the accompanying overpopulation, noise, air and water pollution, job dislocation, decrease in individual privacy, and the adoption of every technological advance without regard to its impact on health and living habits have created additional social and psychological tension.

The stoic followers of the philosopher Zeno believed that humans should be unmoved by passion, should be free from joy and grief, and should submit without complaint to the unavoidable necessities of life. Twenty-three hundred years later, only slight changes in the proposed characteristics of good emotional health have emerged. In other words, society dictates, in general, that emotion should be properly controlled; one should not be overpowered by feelings of joy, grief, fear, or anger. One should be able to take responsibilities and disappointments in stride.

Has man's coping abilities or strategies been equally advanced? Has the structure and function of the biological organism significantly changed? The answer to both questions is no. Even though Athenaeus suggested that no one can afford to be ignorant of medicine and the Stoics desired that lessons in the preservation of tranquility be administered from the earliest age, modern man knows little about the preservation of health, especially that of emotional health. Likewise, very little educational time is spent on the same.

We know, as the Stoics knew, that maintenance of health necessitates some intervention in the stress-arousal cycle. One must diminish the overreaction to environmental stimuli and cool the fires of imagination. To quiet the mind, one must obtain tranquility, but not everyone has the philosophical growth to live a tranquil life, and many psychological traits promote a runaway imagination. The most popular solution is a temporary alteration in one's state of consciousness, or a high.

Being high is a multidimensional state difficult to describe, for it can be viewed solely as a psychological experience, as an increased attention to feeling-experiencing, rather than a doing-planning state. Or it can be described as a physical experience, an altered sensory environment or a breakdown in the normal thought process. Most often it is described in psychophysiological terms as an "egoless state," one in

/hich the environment is perceived as nonthreatening and the ego does not have ɔ be defended. Whatever the description, being high represents a psychophysiologi-al state significantly different from the normal, alert, waking state.

There exists in the mind an automatization of hierarchically ordered psychologi-al "processes," perhaps better thought of as methods of thinking or processing ıformation. These processes conserve attentional energy for maximal efficiency in ᴄhieving the basic goals of the individual in society, i.e., psychological survival of ɴe's personality and physiological survival of the organism (Table 12.1). Under ᵖecial conditions of dysfunction such as in cases of acute psychosis, in some drugged ᵗates, or in some meditative states, the system of automatic thought processing ▸reaks down and permits a less efficient mode of processing in which everyday activi-ᵢes, feeling, or events are perceived differently or shifted more toward perceptual ᵢnd cognitive functioning. This may be thought of as more primitive than the ₐnalytical, abstract, intellectualization that is typical of the normal waking state [2].

ᴦABLE 12.1
ᴦhe normal state

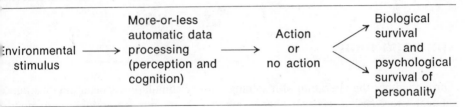

| Environmental stimulus | → | More-or-less automatic data processing (perception and cognition) | → | Action or no action | < | Biological survival and psychological survival of personality |

THE ALTERED STATE

An altered state of consciousness can be induced by various physiological, psycho-logical, or pharmacological maneuvers or agents that alter the enteroreceptive stim-ulation necessary for maintenance of normal waking consciousness. Levels of stimu-lation above or below the optimal range are conducive to producing altered states of consciousness. Examples are:

1. Maneuvers or agents which reduce stimulation and/or motor activity, such as prolonged social and stimulus deprivation, solitary confinement, mystical or transcendental states, passive meditation, floating on water, extreme muscle re-laxation, production of alpha or theta states and some depressant drugs.

2. Maneuvers or agents which increase stimulation and/or motor activity such as brainwashing, revivalistic meetings, ecstatic trances, prolonged vigilance as dur-ing sentry duty, intense mental absorption as in many tasks of reading, writing, or problem-solving, or certain psychedelic or stimulant drugs.

3. Certain somatopsychological factors or alterations in body chemistry such as hypoglycemia, dehydration, sleep deprivation, administration of anesthetic, psy-chedelic, stimulant, or sedative drugs.

Despite the apparent differences among altered states, there are a number of characteristics commonly reported:

1. Disturbed time sense, either a feeling of timelessness (time coming to a stand still) or an acceleration of time.
2. Disturbance in concentration, attention, or memory.
3. Blurred distinctions between cause and effect.
4. A feeling of loss of self-control, or a lessening of inhibitions.
5. A sense of depersonalization.
6. Perceptual distortions, usually with increased visual imagery.
7. A change in the meaning or significance of subjective experiences or ideas.
8. Increased suggestibility.

Some or all of these feelings plus some somatic effects not mentioned constitute the "high" which, as previously mentioned, can be induced by a variety of maneuvers o agents [4].

THE DRUG HIGH

Through either the alteration of incoming sensory stimuli or the deautomatization of thought processes, drugs can change awareness, memory, emotions, and moods. Such alterations give an air of novelty to everyday occurrences, thus changing their significance and one's interest in them. Motivations become obscure and one may begin pondering the significance of an object, feeling, or idea, forgetting that it was previously rendered insignificant. Obligations and goals become obscure and somewhat meaningless, as experiencing the moment becomes extremely pleasurable. The anxiety of passing time is diminished. What is real and important is making sense of the impulses that have the attention of the consciousness. Awareness is heightened, and imagery becomes more stimulating and significant. Touch, taste, and smell are not just stimulators of the senses—their origins become part of the body or mind. The sense of unrealness and the lack of ego involvement is calming, but the learned tendency of the mind to create logic and order often gains awareness, thus creating alterations in moods that oscillate between pleasure and apprehension. At times, goal-directed activity seems alien and the body is only intermittently disturbed by sporadic arousal. Most often the stress of time, goals, and ego are reduced, as are the pressures of everyday existence.

A drug-induced high is often an idyllic experience but one that is not without drawbacks. Chronic use of drugs to obtain an altered state of consciousness tends to develop an unrealistic concept of self and reality that demands an inordinate amount of pleasure from each situation, in which feelings become more important than actions. Happiness is increasingly defined as immediate pleasure with less reference given to delayed gratification. An overemphasis on the feeling world of subective experiences may lead to withdrawal, resulting in self-absorption, selfishness, and a decreased motivation to participate in the search for creative growth experiences.

Intensity of the drug-induced high is dependent on such factors as timing, dosage, purity, setting, state of mind, and motivation, to mention a few. Frustration and disappointment may develop when expectations are not met, and fear, apprehension, and injury can result if the drug is too strong or adulterated. Either way the individual is not in control of the experience; he or she is in a sense imprisoned in an altered state of consciousness until the drug has been metabolized. Often the experience is too intense, too deep, or in a sense too removed from the learning, remembering, processing, "I-Normal" state; thus, little is remembered or learned. In the *Master Game* Robert DeRopp [3] writes that although some transcendence of self is experienced, a drug high is but a glimpse of transcendence. Drugs are uncontrollable; thus, in order to gain inner awareness and to play the master game (searching for metaphysical rewards), one needs all one's thoughts, feelings, and resources.

The passivity of the drug experience is in itself an often-mentioned drawback. Passive experiences in which the individual just rides along, seeing, feeling, and experiencing are somehow not as satisfying as those in which the individual is the active, creative center of the experience. Such activities increase one's feeling of self-esteem, and in a circular pattern increase motivation and readiness for future unknown ventures.

NONDRUG HIGHS

Meditation

The most popular method of getting high or inducing an altered state of consciousness without drugs is through yoga or meditation, which is a form of Raja yoga or yoga of self-realization. Meditation allows one to transcend conscious thought to reach more subtle states of mind, to quiet the mind and the imagination which are sources of stressful arousal. It is a state described as "restful alertness," indicative of the fourth major state of consciousness, just as natural as the other three physiologically defined states: wakefulness, dreaming, and deep sleep. (The five states of consciousness are deep sleep, REM sleep, the awake or "I-Normal" stage, self-transcendence, and cosmic consciousness.) In the Western world its most popular form is transcendental meditation (TM) as taught by Maharishi Mahesh Yogi through an organization called the Students International Meditation Society. The purpose of this discussion, however, is not to judge the value of this particular method of meditation, but to use it as an example, since it is the most popular (350,000 people in the United States have completed the course).

The eight-hour course in transcendental meditation is easy to complete. Two hours of the course are devoted to an introduction and a sales-type lecture on its physiological benefits. Another hour is given to an initiation rite to impress on the student that he or she is following ancient traditions. Finally one is given a mantra, a meaningless word used to focus attention and to aid in clearing the mind of ongoing "story-type" thoughts. The remaining four hours is devoted to practice and discus sions of problems encountered. The goal of meditation is more to quiet the mind and reduce stress arousal than to serve as a substitute for drugs, but there are many similarities and SIMS claims that many drug-users-turned-meditators never return to the use of drugs. Meditation does not produce the sensory depression that drugs do; however, visual imagery is often reported. Meditation is described in terms of awareness of subtle thoughts, energy, and creative intelligence. It is a transcendence of consciousness that enables one to recognize and experience his or her internal flow of energy, creativity, and intelligence. Problems can be seen and attacked on a fundamental level without specific regard to the nature of the problem.

The meditation experience is not as intense as the drug high nor is it as danger- ous or debilitating. The meditator is not trapped in the altered state of consciousness as the drugged person is. By having command over emotions, feelings and memory, more sense can be made out of the experience. Most important, meditation is an active rather than a passive process, one that takes practice and thought. The indi- vidual is left with the feeling of creativity and accomplishment and a more positive feeling about his or her activity.

One problem with meditation is the subjectiveness of the process. Most students simply take for granted that if they do what the instructor says, they are in fact meditating; but many express doubt of obtaining an altered state and like to be tested. Electroencephalographic studies on masters do show that during meditation, slowed brain-wave states are induced. However, little objective data exists on medi- tators with less than a year's experience.

Biofeedback

Another method of aiding one in obtaining slowed brain-wave states is alpha or theta biofeedback. Generally, biofeedback is a system of monitoring bioelectrical signals emitted from the body (internal activity that the individual would not usually be aware of, such as in this case, brain states which are associated with relaxation and calmness) and of transforming that information to visual or auditory signals that allow the individual to become aware of many aspects of his or her state of being. With the proper instrumentation one can be taught rather easily to produce, at will, a state associated with slowed brain waves, below 13 cycles per second. The brain is constantly producing electrical activity that can be measured from the surface of the skull. The usual "nonthinking" wave emitted is a strong, slow wave of between 8 to 13 cycles per second, called an *alpha wave*. When this pattern becomes desynchro- nized in response to stimuli, the *beta wave* pattern emerges and analytic thinking is increased. The beta waves are low-voltage, fast waves of between 14 and 50 cycles per second. Feelings during beta have been described as anticipatory, frustrated, in- vestigative, conceptualizing, and impatient (to mention a few). Alpha has been described as neutral, sluggish, dreamlike, pleasant. Theta, a state characterized by waves slower than alpha, has been described as fuzzy, puzzled, unreal, creative, visionary (Table 12.2).

TABLE 12.2
States of consciousness as determined by brain waves, and feelings often associated with each state [1]

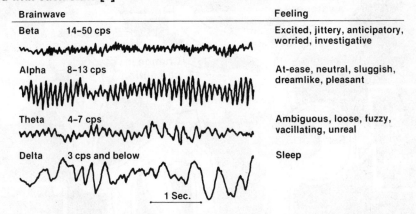

Brainwave		Feeling
Beta	14–50 cps	Excited, jittery, anticipatory, worried, investigative
Alpha	8–13 cps	At-ease, neutral, sluggish, dreamlike, pleasant
Theta	4–7 cps	Ambiguous, loose, fuzzy, vacillating, unreal
Delta	3 cps and below	Sleep

1 Sec.

Researchers and clinicians are using EEG biofeedback to train individuals to produce and maintain slow brain-wave states at will. The motivation varies from the reduction of stress, to "getting high," to increasing creativity. The benefits are similar to those previously listed for meditation, i.e., a production of an altered state of consciousness, an interaction with the interior self, an increased self-awareness, and increased self-control. Like meditation the individual actively produces the state at will and can terminate it instantly, while remaining close to normal thinking consciousness. Unlike meditation, however, the individual knows for sure that an altered brain state does exist. However, biofeedback is only a learning tool. One learns to produce the state and sense its presence, and to reproduce it without the instrument. The sensing is thus transferred to an autosensory system. A drawback to biofeedback is that good instrumentation is expensive. What is available for less than $500 is totally inadequate. Yet, biofeedback has become so popular that those interested can usually search out a research project, counseling center, or clinic that may offer training.

It is extremely difficult to produce a tranquil, altered state of consciousness without drugs, if the brain is being bombarded with stimuli. For example, if muscles are tense, feedback heightens activity of the reticular activating system and cortex activity is increased, further tensing the muscles and creating a positive feedback system which makes relaxation difficult. Slowed brain waves may be impossible if such alpha-blocking activity is not reduced. Techniques of respiration and muscle control are part of many yoga styles and are central to tension control programs such as that of progressive muscle relaxation made famous by Dr. Edmund Jacobson. This system utilizes the inherent autosensory mechanism in muscles first to make one aware of sensations of tension arising within those muscles, and second, to aid in the voluntary control over muscles to reduce that tension. As in meditation the student must be trained in the art of passive concentration so that alertness may be maintained, but that concentration must not itself induce tension and anxiety. Biofeedback clinicians have likewise used the art of passive concentration, but have

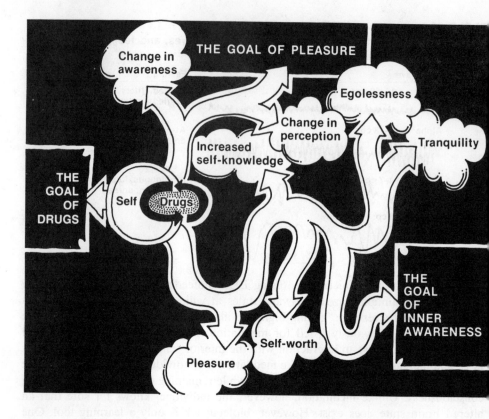

added the electromyograph to allow one to recognize muscle tension and as a teaching aid in the reduction of that tension. Again biofeedback enables more rapid learning through more exact information.

To achieve full relaxation one cannot be apprehensive; one must void one's mind of memories, anticipations, and awareness of pain. Focusing on the muscles or the internal self in general enhances one's awareness of self and enables one to better recognize the influence of thought on feeling and physical reactions. One begins to see the mind and the body as a unit.

SELF-TRANSCENDENCE

Many desire an altered state of consciousness to experience the higher transcendent nature of self generally recognized as the fourth state of consciousness, *self-transcendence*. This feeling has been defined as a state of relative egolessness, free from anxiety and defenses, which allow for expansion of experiences and feelings and for increased knowledge of self. Such states have been described as a high and termed by Maslow [5] as a "peak experience": "the greatest attainment of identity, autonomy or selfhood." Not to be constantly lived in or planned for, peak experiences just happen, seldom to most people and more often to those whose aim is inner awareness. Drugs allow only glimpses, techniques such as meditation and biofeedback promote learning, but self-transcendent peak experiences are part of a life style, or a philosophy of living. Yet the practice of Creative Psychology (one of its many homonyms) is based on the premise that one can change one's level of being and level of awareness, and increase the frequency of peak experiences [3].

To Maslow, a person in a peak experience takes on, at least temporarily, some of the characteristics of his often described "self-actualized" individual: "Not only are these his happiest moments, but they are also moments of greatest maturity, individualism, fulfillment—in a word his healthiest moments" [5]. In this context self-actualization is not an all-or-none phenomenon, but a spurt in which the powers of a person are unified and integrated. Parts of the self are functioning harmoniously and not laboring in restraint, not wasting energies on indecision. A reduction in inhibition allows a more spontaneous natural expression of self and one becomes the active, creative center of activity. In the eyes of others, a more reliable, trustworthy, and less defensive posture invites additional opportunities; this in turn promotes development of self-esteem which increases adequacy of coping responses and assures increased frequencies of peak experiences.

Unfortunately, there are no substances or simple techniques to assure attainment of such a state, but volumes have been written on successful and unsuccessful pursuits. One first needs philosophical and psychological growth and development (which provide realization and motivation), good teachers, and literary guidance. (It is hoped that the readings listed at the end of this chapter will provide a beginning for such literary pursuit.)

SUMMARY

One might view the highs discussed in this chapter as a hierarchy. On the low end are drug-induced highs. Except for potential physical dangers, side effects, etc., and a lack of control over them, they may be better than no high at all; for drugs afford glimpses of self-transcendence, moments of egolessness; and if one is not deluded by pleasurable feelings into thinking that drugs are learning and fulfilling experiences, they may even provide motivation for a continued search.

Next on the hierarchy of highs are what one might consider the techniques. These are a more positive approach than drugs, not only because they are less dangerous, more socially acceptable, and more controllable, but also because they are active and creative, and require and promote self-control and self-discipline. These are learning exercises which, if mastered, provide the foundation and motivation needed to reeducate one's self toward positive coping and positive health.

Still higher is the conscious high or peak experience: conscious self-transcendence, egolessness to the extent that ego is strengthened so that its boundaries are infinitely extended and unshakable. It is a needless state because needs are fulfilled. It is a higher state because such states are integrated with ongoing life, and provide benefits to society and mankind in general. Considering average ambitions, it is almost impossible to reach such states without social goal fulfillment which satisfies most lower-need gratifications that can be bought with money (safety and physiological needs). When these are fulfilled, within reason, a healthy personality strives toward gratification of meta needs.

Many philosophers believe that at the pinnacle of the hierarchy lies a fifth level of consciousness, "cosmic consciousness," or a state of oneness with the universe. This state defies a brief description because if it exists, it is obtainable only after a lifetime of training and complete attainment of the fourth state. Drugs, meditation, or zazen may provide either glimpses of or temporary presence in such a state which may be uninhabited at least in typical Western philosophy.

REFERENCES

1. Brown, B. B., *New Mind, New Body*. New York: Harper & Row, 1974.
2. Deikman, A. J., "Deautomatization and the Mystic Experience," in C. T. Tart, ed., *Altered States of Consciousness*. New York: Doubleday, 1969.
3. DeRopp, R. S., *The Master Game*. New York: Dell, 1968.
4. Ludwig, A. M., "Altered States of Consciousness," in C. T. Tart, ed., *Altered States of Consciousness*. New York: Doubleday, 1969.
5. Maslow, A. H., *Toward a Psychology of Being*. New York: Reinhold, 1968.

SUGGESTED READING

Aaronson, Bernard, and Humphrey Osmond, *Psychedelics*. New York: Doubleday, 1970.

Boisen, A., *The Exploration of the Inner World*. New York: Harper & Row, 1962.

Brena, Steven F., *Yoga and Medicine*. Baltimore: Penguin Books, 1972.

Cochrane, R., "Values as Correlates of Deviancy," *British Journal of Social and Clinical Psychology*, 13(3):257–267, September 1974.

Hoffer, Eric, *The Ordeal of Change*. New York: Harper & Row, 1963.

Maslow, Abraham H., *Religion, Values and Peak-Experiences*. New York: Viking Press, 1970.

Mesthene, Emmanuel G., *Technological Change*. New York: New American Library, 1970.

Mishria, Rammurti, *Yoga*. New York: Lancer Books, 1959.

Robbins, Jhan, and David Fisher, *Tranquility Without Pills*. New York: Wyden, 1972.

Rogers, Carl, *On Becoming a Person*. Boston: Houghton Mifflin, 1961.

Russell, Bertrand, *The Conquest of Happiness*. New York: Liveright, 1958.

Szasz, Thomas, *Ceremonial Chemistry*. Garden City, N.J.: Anchor Press, 1974.

Tart, C. T., ed., *Altered States of Consciousness*. New York: Doubleday, 1969.

White, John, ed., *The Highest State of Consciousness*. New York: Doubleday, 1972.

GLOSSARY

Abstinence syndrome	Physiological and psychological symptoms that result from abrupt withdrawal from depressants; intense manifestation of the stress reaction
Abuse	Use improperly
Acid	LSD (lysergic acid diethylamide)
Acidhead	Chronic user of LSD
Acute	Of short duration and severe
Addiction	A state resulting from regular use of drugs (especially depressants) that create physical dependence
All lit up	Under the influence of a drug
Amine	A substance having an NH_2 group in its chemical structure
Amytal	A barbiturate of intermediate action
Analgesic	A pain-relieving chemical
Anesthetic	A chemical substance producing a loss of feeling and relief from pain
Antagonistic	Having or producing opposite effects
Antidepressant	A chemical that counteracts depressed feelings
Around the turn	Having passed through the worst part of withdrawal
Artillery	Apparatus for injecting drugs
Bad trip	Unpleasant experience, usually caused by panic reaction after taking a drug
Bag	A small quantity of drugs, usually heroin
Bagman	Small-time drug supplier
Bamboo	Opium pipe
Bang	Inject, or to get a thrill from injection
Bar	A solid block of marijuana with sugar or Coca-Cola to make it stick together
Barbs	Barbiturates
Belly habit	Opiate addiction (one of the first signs of withdrawal from opiates is stomach cramps)
Benny	Benzedrine
Benny jag	High on Benzedrine
Big chief	Mescaline
Big D	LSD
Big John	The police
Big man	High-level pusher
Black beauties	Biphetamine
Blackout	Temporary loss of memory
Blue devils	Amytal
Blue velvet	A paregoric antihistamine mixture

Burned	Got phony drugs
Burned out	Sclerosis of veins from puncturing
Bust	Drug raid
Buttons	Usable part of the peyote cactus
C	Cocaine
Candy	Barbiturates
Cap	Capsule of a drug, usually heroin
Cartwheels	Amphetamine tablets scored into quarters
Chippying or chippy	Irregular drug use
Christmas trees	Dexamyl
Chronic	Of long duration
Coast	Euphoric nodding state of a heroin high
Coke	Cocaine
Cold turkey	Withdrawal without the tapering-off process
Coming down	The period when the effects of a drug, especially LSD, begin to wear off
Connect	Find a source and buy drugs
Cooker	Spoon or bottle cap to mix and heat heroin for injection
Co-pilots	Amphetamines
Crash	Fall asleep after a prolonged high
Crystal	Methamphetamine
Cube	Cube of sugar containing LSD
Cut	Dilute drugs, usually with milk sugar
Dabble	Use drugs irregularly
Dealer	Seller or pusher of drugs
Dexie	Dexedrine, an amphetamine
DMT	Dimethyltryptamine; similar in structure to psilocin, but altered synthetically
DOM	Dimethoxymethylamphetamine (STP)
Double trouble	Tuinal, a barbiturate
Downers	Barbiturates, tranquilizers, alcohol, any depressant
Dried out	Withdrawn from drugs completely
Drivers or truckdrivers	Amphetamines
Drop	Swallow, take orally
Dynamite	High-grade heroin, sometimes mixed with cocaine
Euphoria	Exaggerated sense of well-being
Experience	An LSD-type trip
Eye openers	Amphetamines
Factory	Place for the manufacture of illicit drugs

Fives	5-milligram tablets, usually amphetamines
Fix	A shot of narcotics
Flake	Cocaine
Flash	Sudden rush of euphoria after injection of speed or heroin
Flea powder	Inferior or phony drugs
Freakout	A bad experience, or temporary psychotic reaction
Fruit salad	Game of taking many different pills
Fuzz	The police
Gassing	Sniffing the fumes from gasoline
Glow	High, euphoria
Gold leaf	High-grade marijuana
Goof ball	Barbiturate
Goofers	Doriden
Grass	Marijuana
Grasshopper	One who uses marijuana
H	Heroin
Habituation	Compulsive drug use
Hallucinations	Perceptions with no external reality
Hard stuff	Opiates, heroin
Hash	Hashish, pure resin from the cannabis plant; most potent source of THC
Hay	Marijuana
Hearts	Amphetamine tablets so shaped
Heat	Police investigation
Hemp	Marijuana
Hooked	Addicted
Horse	Heroin
Jag	Intoxication
Joint	Marijuana cigarette
Jolly beans	Pep pills
Jones	Heroin withdrawal
Joy-pop or skin-pop	Inject drugs under the skin
Juice	Liquor
Junk	Narcotics
Junkie	One who uses narcotics regularly, usually addicted
Kick	Break the drug habit
Kilo	A kilogram (2.2 pounds) brick of marijuana
L	LSD-25
Lemonade	Poor-grade heroin

Lid	A street measure of marijuana, about an ounce; makes into about 40 marijuana cigarettes, depending on how clean it is
M	Morphine
Mainline	Inject drugs into a vein
Maintaining	Keeping a certain level of drug habit
Man	The police
Manicure	Marijuana of high grade; or (as a verb) to remove the stems and seeds from marijuana leaves
Matchbox	A street measure of marijuana, about 0.2 ounce; makes into about 6 to 7 marijuana cigarettes
Mescal	Peyote
Meth	Methamphetamine
Mexican brown	Good grade of marijuana from Mexico
Mike	Microgram (usually of LSD); equals one-millionth of a gram
Miltown	Meprobamate, a tranquilizer
Nalline	A semisynthetic derivative of morphine, Nalorphine hydrochloride
Narc	Federal narcotics officer
Nembies	Nembutal, a barbiturate
Nickel bag	$5 worth of drugs
O	Opium
OD	Overdose
On	Under the influence of drugs
On the street	Out of jail
Oranges	Dexedrine tablets
O.T.C.	Over-the-counter, nonprescription drugs
Pad	Room or house; may imply place for taking drugs
Panic	Anxiety over a shortage of drugs on the market
Paper	Paper for writing prescriptions
Peachies	Benzedrine in tablet form
Pep pills	Amphetamines
P.G.	Paregoric
Phenos	Phenobarbital
Pillhead	Person using amphetamines or barbiturates
Pink ladies	Seconal, barbiturate
Pot	Marijuana
Psychotogenic	Having the power to produce psychosis
Psychotomimetic	Having the power to mimic psychosis
Putting the bean	Begging for narcotics

Quarter bag	1 ounce of marijuana, sold for $25
Rainbow	Tuinal capsule, a barbiturate
Rap	Communicate, speak with rapport
Red devils, red birds, or reds	Seconal, a barbiturate
Reefer	Marijuana cigarette
Roach	Marijuana cigarette butt
Roach holder	Matchbook cover, toothpick, hairpin, or other device used to hold the last bit of a marijuana cigarette so it can be smoked
Rope	Marijuana
Rush	Sudden onset of euphoria
Sam	Narcotics agent of the federal government
Scars	Needle marks
Score	Find and buy drugs
Seccy or seggy	Seconal, a barbiturate
Seed	Marijuana cigarette butt
Setting	Proper environment to take drugs, especially hallucinogens
Shoot up	Inject drugs
Shooting gallery	A safe place to shoot up
Sitter	A person who is experienced in the use of LSD and aids someone else through the experience
Scag	Heroin
Smack	Heroin
Sniffing	Inhaling toxic vapors or snow
Snow	Cocaine
Source	Steady supplier of drugs
Speed	Methamphetamine
Speed freak	Habitual user of speed
Square	Nonuser
Stash	A hidden supply of drugs
Stoned	Under the influence of drugs
STP	Dimethoxymethylamphetamine (DOM), a synthetic hallucinogen; STP may stand for the motor oil additive "scientifically treated petroleum" or "serenity, tranquility, and peace"
Street, on the street	Out searching for drugs
Strung out	Being addicted
Sweet Lucy	Resinous part of marijuana dissolved in wine

all	Being high or stoned
aste	Small amount of drugs
exas tea	Marijuana
HC	Tetrahydrocannabinol, the active ingredient in marijuana and hashish that causes psychogenic reactions
ingle	Rush or high feeling
ooies	Tuinal, a barbiturate
rip or tripping out	An experience with LSD or other hallucinogens
urned off	Withdrawn from drugs
urned on	High on drugs
ncle	Federal narcotics officer
p	High on drugs
ppers	Amphetamines or other stimulants
asted	Passed out from overintoxication
eed	Marijuana
hites	Benzedrine in pill form
ired	High on drugs, especially amphetamines
ellow jackets	Nembutal, a barbiturate
en	Strong desire for drugs

INDEX

Abstinence syndrome, 5, 144
  and alcohol, 52
Accidental death, 140–141
Acetaldehyde, 39, 121
Acetaminophen, 183
Acetic acid, 39
Acetylcholine, 19, 127, 166, 179
Acetylmethadol, 167
Acetylsalicylic acid, 180, 182–183
Acne preparations, 186
ACTH, 166
Addict, 161–164
Addiction, 4; *see also* Physical dependence,
    Psychological dependence
  to alcohol, 52
  to heroin, 161–164
Addictive personality, 52–53, 161–162, 164
Adrenal glands, 80, 104, 127
Advertising
  of cigarettes, 123
  of OTC drugs, 178, 188
Alcohol, 32–60
  absorption of, 34, 36, 44–45
  as aphrodisiac, 46
  blood alcohol concentration, 43–44
  body temperature, 45
  caloric value, 38–39
  dependence on, 33, 52
  depressant action of, 34–36
  drinking population, 48–49
  and driving skill, 43
  effect on brain, 34
  fetal effects, 45–46
  metabolism, 38–39, 40, 42
  nutritional value of, 37–38, 52
  physical effects of, 44
  physiological tolerance to, 33–34
  proof-percentage, 41–43, 44
  psychological effects of, 44
  terminology, 60
  toxicosis, 36
Alcohol treatment, 53–57
Alcoholics Anonymous, 55–56
Alcoholism, 48–57
  causative factors, 52–53
  phases of, 50–52

Alienation, 10, 12, 70
Alka-Plus, 183
Altered states of consciousness, 210–218
  drug high, 212–213
  nondrug high, 213–218
Aluminum hydroxide, 186
Alveoli, 129
Ambar, 199
Amobarbital, 199
Amphetamines, 23, 25, 104–117
  absorption of, 104
  abuse of, 109–112
  action on central nervous system, 24, 25
  and athletic performance, 107–109
  dangers of, 109–112
  as diet aids, 107
  dosage, 106
  and driving skills, 109
  history of, 104
  identification, 105
  laws concerning, 106, 199, 201
  medical use, 106
  and mental performance, 109
  misuse of, 107–109
  pharmacological effects, 104
  physiological effects, 104
  pleasure, 110
  and pleasure centers, effect on, 23
  psychosis, 112
  psychotomimetic, 94–95
  and satiety, effect on, 23, 107
  studying, 109
  terminology, 116–117
  toxicity, 112
  use of, 106–109
Amytal, 139, 199
Anacin, 183
Analgesics, 182–185
Antabuse, 55
Antacid, 186–187
Antibiotics, 4
Anticholinergic action, 179
Antihistamines, 179, 180
Anti-inflammatory action of aspirin, 185
Antiobesity preparations, 185–186
Antipyretic action of aspirin, 185

Aphrodisiac, alcohol as, 46
Arousal, *see* Reticular activating system
Aspergum, 183
Aspirin, 182–184
Association area of cortex, 26
Athletic performance, effects of amphetamines on, 107–109
Atropine, 180
Axon, 18

Bad trip, 85–87
Bamadex, 199
Barbiturates, 136–150, 155
  abuse of, 142–147
  history of, 136
  identification, 139
  laws governing use of, 201
  medical uses, 136
  misuse, dangers of, 138–141
  sleep patterns, 138–140
  treatment of withdrawal from, 145–147
Belladonna alkaloids, 179, 180
Benzedrine, 104, 199
Benzocaine preparations, 186
Bhang, 65
Biofeedback, 55, 214–216
Blackouts, 50–51
Blood alcohol content, 43
Blood-brain barrier, 80
Body temperature
  and alcohol, 45
  and aspirin, 185
  and LSD, 81, 95
Boggs Act, 199
Boredom, 7
Bouton, 18
Brain, 21–28
Brain function, 21–28
Brainstem, 21–28
  and alcohol, 36
  and LSD, 81
British system, 165
Bromide, 136
Brompheriramine, 180
Bronchitis, 130
Bufferin, 183
Bureau of Narcotics and Dangerous Drugs, 106, 198

Caffeine, 41, 113, 152, 186
California v. *Woody,* 202
Calories, in alcoholic beverages, 38–39
Cancer, lung, 128–129, 131
Cannabis, *see* Marijuana
Cannabis sativa, 64
Carcinogens, 120
Central nervous system
  effect of alcohol on, 33
  effect of sedative hypnotics on, 137

Cerebellum, 26
Cerebral cortex, 26–27, 81, 137, 154
  association areas, 26
  sensory areas, 26
Charas, 65
Chaser, 183
Chlordiazepoxide, 139
Chlorpromazine, 86
Chromosomes, effect of LSD on, 87–88
Cigarettes, *see* Smoking
Cilia, 120–122
Cirrhosis, 47–48
Civil commitment to drug rehabilitation, 170–171
Claviceps purpurea, 80
Cocaine, 113–114, 199
Codeine, 154, 199
Co-Gel, 183
Commission on Marijuana and Drug Abuse 63–64, 201
Compoz, 179, 182
Comprehensive Drug Abuse Prevention and Control Act, 160, 198–199, 201, 202
Conformity, *see* Peer pressure
Convulsions, 86, 145
Coordination, 26
Cope, 183
Creativity, 8
  and LSD, 90
  and mescaline, 90
Criminalization, 194
Curiosity, 6, 24, 72
Cyclazocine, 167

Daytop Village, 169
Demerol, 199
Dendrite, 18
Dependence, *see* Physical dependence, Psychological dependence
Depression, mental, 20, 106
Desoxyn, 199
DET (diethyltryptamine), 94, 199
Dexamyl, 199
Dexedrine, 104, 199
Diazepam, 96, 139, 147
Diet pills, 107
Dilaudid, 154, 199
Dipherhydramine, 180
DMT (dimethyltryptamine), 94, 199
DOM, *see* STP
Dopamine, 19, 104
Doriden, 139, 146, 199
Drug, definition of, 2
Drug abuse
  definition of, 2
  history of, 3
  motivation for, 5–13
Drug Enforcement Administration, 160, 198
Drug entry into the United States, 155–156

rug misuse
  definition of, 2
  history of, 3
rug use, definition of, 2
rug-using population, 6
  and alcohol, 48–49
  and heroin, 159, 161
  and marijuana, 71–73
DT's (delirium tremens), 52
Durham-Humphrey Act, 201

Ego boundary, 82
Emotions, see Hypothalamus, Limbic system
Emphysema, 129–130
Energy, 39
Epinephrine, 108, 113
Equanil, 137, 139, 199
Ergot alkaloids, 80
Escape drinking, 50
Ethanol, 33
Ethchlorynol, 139
Euphoria, 3, 5, 95, 110, 154, 181
Excedrin, 183
Exercise, in treatment of alcoholism, 55

Federal Food and Drug Administration, 188
  and laws governing OTC drugs, 187–188
Felony, 202
Fermentation, 3
Fetus
  effect of alcohol on, 45–46
  effect of LSD on, 88
  effect of smoking on, 130–131
Flashbacks
  from LSD use, 86–87
  from marijuana use, 69
Food, Drug, and Cosmetic Act, 187, 201
Formaldehyde, 121

Gamma amino butyric acid, 19
Ganja, 65
Glucose preparations, 186
Glue, 204–205
Glutethimide, 136, 139, 146
Goal fulfillment, see Philosophy of drug use
Group pressure, see Peer pressure
Group therapy
  and alcoholism, 55
  and heroin use, 168–171
  and smoking, 126

Habituation, 4
Halfway houses, 169–170
Hallucinogens, 80–102; see also LSD
  purity, 85
  relative potency, 92
  synthetic, 94–95
  terminology, 101–102
Hangover, 40

Harrison Narcotic Act, 113, 158, 192, 196, 197
Hashish, 65
Heart disease, 127–128
Hepatitis, 112
Heroin, 152–171, 199; see also Opiates
Histamine, 179
Homatropine, 180
Homeostasis, 23–24
Hunger, 23
Hydrogen cyanide, 121
Hyperkinetic activity, 25
Hypodermic syringe, 3
Hypothalamus, 23–24, 95, 110

Identity, 12
Inhibition, 18, 26, 34
Intoxication
  barbiturate, 141
  legal, 43
  marijuana, 71–72
  peyote, 93

Jones Act, 32
Juveniles, and the law, 205–206

Laudanum, 154
Law, drugs and the, 192–208
  classification of drugs, 198–199
  Commissioner of Narcotics, 196
  and the Constitution, 193
  contempt for, 193–194
  and drug abuse, effect on, 194–196
  minors, 205–206
  model glue, 204–205
  need for, 192
  philosophical basis, 192–196
  possession, 204, 205
  regulation of social conduct, 192–196
  religion, 202
  search and seizure, 204
Laxatives, 186
Leary, Timothy, 83, 197, 202
Levallorphan, 155
Librium, 137, 139, 182
Limbic system, 27–28, 81, 95, 110, 138
Lobeline, 126
LSD (lysergic acid diethylamide), 80–90, 199
  absorption of, 80–81
  and chromosomes, 87–88
  chronic psychosis, 87
  concentration in brain, 80–81
  creativity, 90
  dangers of, 85–86
  dosage, 81
  flashbacks, 86–87
  history, 80
  legal aspects, 199, 201, 202
  neurochemical action of, 81–82

LSD (*cont.*)
  perception, 82
  pharmacology of, 80–81
  physiological effects of, 81
  psychological effects of, 87
  psychotherapy, 89
  purity, 85
  religion, 82–85
  tolerance, 81
  trip, 82
  use of in treatment of alcoholism, 55
Luminal, 136
Lung cancer, 128–129, 131
Lysergic acid, 80; *see also* LSD

Maalox, 183
Magnesium, 186
Mainlining, 155
Maintenance programs, 165–171
Marijuana, 62–77, 199
  and crime, 200
  dosage, 69
  history of, 66
  legalization of, 63–64
  long-term effects, 67–69
  perception distortion, 71
  personality characteristics of users, 70
  physical effects of, 66–69
  population using, 71–73
  potency, 65
  psychosis, 71
  psychosocial effects of, 70–73
  terminology, 76–77
Marijuana Tax Act, 62, 197, 200
Maslow, A. H., 8, 9, 72
May, R., 12
Measurin, 183
Medicine, 2, 3
Meditation, 213
Medulla oblongata, 22
Menstruation, and use of aspirin, 183
Meperidine, 154
Meprobamate, 139, 146
Mescaline, 92–93, 199
Mesencephalon, 22
Metabolism, of alcohol, 38–39, 40, 42
Methadone, 154, 155, 199
Methadone maintenance, 165–167
Methamphetamine, 104, 110
Methapyrilene, 180
Methaqualone, 136, 139, 199
Methedrine, 199
Methyl salicylate, 180
Methylcellulose, 185
Methyprylon, 139
Mexican drugs, 153
Midol, 183
Miltown, 137, 139, 146, 199
Morphine, 3, 152, 154, 155, 199
Motivation for drug use, 5–13

Motor cortex, 26
Mylanta, 183
Mysticism, and use of LSD, 82–85

Nalorphine, 155, 168
Naloxone, 155, 168
Narcolepsy, 106
Narcotic Addict Rehabilitation Act, 194, 19
Narcotic Drug Import and Export Act, 198
Narcotics Control Act, 198
Narcotics Manufacturing Act, 198, 199
National Organization for the Reform of
    Marijuana (NORML), 64
Native American Church, 9, 93, 202
Nembutal, 139, 146
Nerve cell, 18–21
Nerve impulse, transmission of, 18–20
Nervous system, 18–28
    effect of LSD on, 80–81
    effect of sedatives on, 137
Neurohormonal transmitters, 19
Nicotine, 112, 121–122; *see also* Smoking
    absorption of, 127
    drug effects of, 127–128
Nitrazepam, 140
Nitrous oxide, 96
Noludar, 139
Nonprescription drugs, 5, 178–190
    analgesics, 182–185
    antacids, 186–187
    dangers of, 178
    drug culture and, 178, 188–189
    effectiveness of, 178, 187–188
    regulation of, 187–188
    sleep aids, 179–181
    stimulants, 179–180
    tranquilizers, 181–182
Nonsmoker, 120
Norepinephrine, 19, 24, 108, 110, 143, 144
Nutrition, in alcohol, 37, 38, 52
Nytol, 179

Opiate antagonists, 167–168
Opiates, 152–175
    addict, 161–164
    addiction, 158–161
    administration, 155
    availability, 158
    cost, 152–153
    halfway houses, 169–170
    harvest of, 152–153
    history of, 3, 152, 156–160
    laws, 158–159
    legislative programs, 170–171
    maintenance programs, 165–171
    medical use of, 154
    and the military, 155, 158
    and organized crime, 160
    overdose, 155
    pharmacological effects, 154–155

physical dependence, 161–164
preparation, 152
purity, 152–153
rehabilitation, cost of, 153
smoking, 155, 156
Synanon, 168–169
terminology, 174–175
trade routes, 155–156
treatment of addiction to, 164–171
withdrawal, 155, 164
Opium, 3, 152, 199
Overdose, of amphetamines, 112
Over-the-counter drugs, see Nonprescription
    drugs

Pain centers, 23
Panic reaction, in LSD use, 85–87
Paranoia, 111–112
Paregoric, 154, 199
PCP, 95–96
Peer pressure, 11, 72, 122
Penicillin, 4
Pentazocine, 168
Pentobarbital, see Nembutal
Personality disturbance, 52–53; see also
    Addictive personality
Peyote, 92–93, 199
Peyote cactus, 92
Pheniramine, 180
Phenobarbital, 146, 199
Phenols, 120
Philosophy of drug use, 210–218
Physical dependence, 5, 33
    on alcohol, 52
    on barbiturates, 142–145
    on heroin, 161–164
Placidyl, 139
Pleasure, 7, 72; see also Euphoria
Pleasure centers, 23
Poisoning, salicylate, 183
Pons, 22
Postsynaptic membrane, 19
Pregnancy
    and alcohol, 45–46
    and LSD use, 87–88
    and smoking, 130–131
Preludin, 199
Prescriptions, 137, 199
Presynaptic membrane, 19
Prohibition, 32–33, 62
Proposition 19 (California Marijuana
    Initiative), 64
Psilocin, 93–94
Psilocybin, 93–94
Psychedelic therapy, 89
Psychoanalysis, and alcoholism, 54
Psychological dependence
    on alcohol, 53
    on heroin, 161–164
    on marijuana, 70

on sedatives, 142
on smoking, 124
Psycholytic therapy, 89
Psychosis, 211–212
    amphetamine, 111, 112
    LSD, 87
    marijuana, 71
Psychosomatic illness, 24
Psychotherapy with LSD, 55, 89
Pure Food and Drug Act, 158, 187, 196

Quiet Nite, 179
Quietran, 179
Quinine, 153

RAS, see Reticular activating system
Real Sleep, 179
Recreational drugs, 7
Rehabilitation
    of alcoholics, 53–57
    of heroin addicts, 164–171
Religion, 202
    and LSD use, 82–85
Religious experience, see Spiritualism
REM (rapid eye movement) sleep, 138
Reserpine, 137
Respiratory center, 22
Reticular activating system, 24–25, 110, 137
Reward centers, see Hypothalamus, Limbic
    system
Ritalin, 199

Salicylamide, 179, 180
Salicylic acid, 180, 182–185
Satiety centers, 23
Schizophrenia, 89
Scopolamine, 180, 181
Seconal, 139, 199
Sedative hypnotics, 25, 136–137; see also
    Barbiturates
Sedatives, 25, 136–150, 155; see also
    Barbiturates
    dangers of, 138–145
    over-the-counter, 179–182
    terminology, 150
Self-actualization, see Philosophy of drug use
Self-insight, 9, 55, 89, 125
Self-medication, 178
Self-transcendence, 9, 216–217
Serotonin, 19, 81, 143
Sexual behavior
    effect of alcohol on, 46–47
    effect of amphetamines on, 110
Sleep aids, 179–181
Sleep Eze, 179
Sleep patterns, alteration of, 138–140
Sleep Tabs, 179
Sleeping pills, see Sedatives, Barbiturates
Smokers, types of, 124
"Smoker's cough," 121

Smoking, 120–134; *see also* Nicotine
  bronchitis, 130
  cessation programs, 125–127
  emphysema, 129–130
  health consequences of, 127–131
  heart disease, 127–128
  heroin, 155, 156
  lung cancer, 128–129, 131
  motivation for, 122–125
  nicotine effects, 127–128
  and pregnancy, 130–131
  psychological factors, 122–125
  and ulcers, 131
Sobering-up process, 41
Social drinking, 49, 50
Solonaceae, 180
Sominex, 179
Special Action Office for Drug Abuse
    Prevention, 160
"Speed," 104
Spiritualism, 82–85
Stimulants, 104–114, 185–186; *see also*
    specific drug name
Stimulus relay, 22–23
STP, 94–95
Stress reaction, 104
Strychnine, 152
Suicide, 140–141
Sulfa drugs, 4
Synanon, 12, 164, 168–169
Synapse, 18
Synthetic hallucinogens, 94–95
Synthetic narcotics, 154, 155

Tar, cigarette, 120, 128
Technology, 3
Temperature regulation, by aspirin, 185
Teratogenic effects, 67
  of LSD, 87–88
Tetrahydrocannabinol (THC), 65, 199
Thalamus, 22–23, 95, 110
Thorazine, 137
Thought processes, 26–27

Tobacco, 120–122
Tolerance
  to alcohol, 33, 51
  to amphetamines, 110
  to barbiturates, 142–145
  to hallucinogens, 81, 93, 94
Tranquets, 179
Tranquilizers, 4, 137–138, 139, 179, 181–18
Tranquizine, 179
Treatment
  alcoholism, 53–57
  barbiturate addiction, 145–146
  heroin addiction, 164–171
Tuinal, 139, 199
Turkish opium, 160

Ulcers, 186
  and smoking, 131
Uniform Narcotic Drug Act, 200
United States v. *Kuch,* 202

Vaccine, 4
Valium, 137, 139
Veronal, 136
Vesicles, *see* Nerve cell
Violence, 111–112
Vital centers, 22
Vitamins, 54
Volstead Act, 32

Wakefulness, 24, 25, 211
Weight control, 107, 185–186
White House Conference on Narcotics and
    Drug Abuse, 201
Withdrawal, 5
  from alcohol, 52
  from barbiturates, 145–146
  from heroin, 155, 164
  from marijuana, 67

Yablonski, L., 84
Youth culture, 8, 10, 72, 136